Bedside

Nurses, Miracles, and Medical Breakthroughs

Phyllis Heintz

PLATYPUS
PUBLISHING

1st edition 2025
ISBN: 978-1-965016-47-3

Contents

Dedication

To Chuck and Laura. Their enduring love and unwavering belief in me made this work possible.

To Brian, Anthony, and families. Their love and delightful children are precious gifts. One of my greatest joys is being called Aunt Phyllis.

To Sandra, my muse. Her inspiration and support were a guiding light throughout this journey.

To Eileen. Her invaluable insights brought this book to life.

To Harold and Phyllis Heintz. Their love, devotion, and guidance profoundly shaped my life.

Prologue

Such a meaningful milestone—the last class of students I had admitted as Chair, now graduating, marks the end of an era not only for those students but for the program and me. I recently retired as the Chair of the California State University Bakersfield, Department of Nursing. I've seen the students transition from eager learners to capable nurses ready to make a difference. Being here to celebrate their achievement is a full-circle moment, especially as they enter my beloved profession.

I was honored they asked me to be the Inspirational Speaker at their Pinning ceremony and wanted to hear stories about my career. It is a testament to my impact on these students and the profession. Sharing my career adventures with them offers an inspiring perspective, especially as they're about to embark on their nursing journeys. They are eager to learn from someone who lives and loves the profession, having navigated the diverse paths nursing can take. I ponder the dozens of messages I could share with them around the central themes—resilience, perseverance, adaptability, and compassion—that guided my career.

I am anxious about giving the speech and spent a great deal of time practicing it. I selected stories to convey the depth of my experience to inspire them as they step into the profession. I am the inspirational speaker, so I must be passionate for the graduates as well as the family and friends attending the ceremony. Capturing fifty years of nursing into one impactful talk is both challenging and rewarding. Throughout my career I found creative ways to refresh my practice, embrace new roles, and stay inspired amidst all the changes in healthcare.

My demanding career strained under forces within healthcare settings beyond my control. Those forces influenced the never-ending tension between the care I could provide and my job satisfaction. Nurses enter the profession to provide quality care which is jeopardized from reduced staffing levels because of lower hospital reimbursements. Increased nurse workloads adversely impacts patient outcomes. Nurse burnout and reduced job satisfaction are collateral damage. I call this phenomenon of balancing hospital finances with adequate nurse staffing levels to provide safe, quality patient centered care, *The Great Tension*. I tried my best to prepare my students for practice in this environment.

On the day of Pinning, I arrive at the venue, greeted by beaming graduates. They excitedly celebrate their achievement with their loved ones...and me. Hugs and laughter flow around me. The graduates dance down the aisle to *I Gotta Feeling* by the Black-Eyed Peas for their Processional. I smile, admiring their imagination.

As I give the speech, I glance out at the graduates. They are engaged, at least in the first five rows. The bright lights make anything past the first five rows of most venues a dark blur. They give me a standing ovation and I feel good about my delivery. As I return to my seat, I ponder the final remarks of my speech:

It was a privilege *to stand beside each of you as you embark on your nursing career.*

To be honest, I am envious. I would love to be in the seat next to you right now. Fifty years is not nearly long enough to explore all the nursing profession offers.

In closing, I want to leave you with some last thoughts.

Don't settle.

Don't settle professionally or personally.

You deserve the best in life.

You deserve a family that supports you as you live a wholehearted life.

You deserve a practice environment that allows you to give your patients the best care.

You deserve the chance to create an intriguing and meaningful career filled with purpose.

You *will make a difference.*

As the ceremony progresses, it dawns on me that my speech is as much about advising myself as it is about advising the students. I *do* deserve the best life has to offer me. That includes a retirement as meaningful as my career. After the ceremony, I am congratulating our new nurses when I turn to see a tall, slender, older woman earnestly smiling at me.

"Dr. Heintz, may I touch you?" she asks. I struggle to make out her features as the sun behind her blurs my vision. She is wearing a white lace sheath dress and repeats her request to touch me. Dumbfounded, I offer my right arm. She reverently touches it. "Dr. Heintz, I loved your speech and wish my granddaughters could have heard it. I have four granddaughters who are nurses."

I thank her for her kind comments and before we could talk further, she disappears into the crowd. I am distracted from finding her as students appear wanting photos and conversation. Her evaporating into the crowd makes the mysterious woman in the white lace dress even more curious. I don't know if she was a vision or an earthly angel. This chance encounter with her is a moment of grace to fully appreciate this occasion's magic and opens my heart to the wonder of this day. Peace washed over me.

Don't settle. I deserve the best a wholehearted life has to offer.

That means it is time to stop settling for an uninspired retired life. I had imagined days filled with exciting explorations, which they were, but those days were spent *listening* to other people's accomplishments. Retirement for me is about actively pursuing my passions on my terms, just as I did in nursing. I vow to embrace this next phase with curiosity, setting new goals to transform it into a thrilling new chapter of exploration.

In this book I capture the essence of nursing and the tugging urgency for a renewed passion for the field in the face of mounting tensions in the profession. I invite readers to walk along with me as I relive the career of a lifetime. My firsthand insights into nurses' unique position in witnessing and supporting medical miracles—and the profound connections formed along the way—will resonate with newcomers and experienced nurses. Anecdotes about innovations I witnessed firsthand show these "miracles" in action. By weaving in the broader American medical innovation story, I am honoring the profession and inviting readers from all walks of life to see nursing as a critical part of societal progress. These are powerful illustrations of nurses' vital role in these pivotal moments.

> **"To know even one life has breathed easier because you have lived. This is to have succeeded."**
>
> —— Ralph Waldo Emerson

Part I

1969 – A Pivotal Year in Medicine

Opening Thoughts

The astronauts' landing on the moon on July 20, 1969, was a watershed moment for our country. Like other Americans, my brother, Chuck, and I were fascinated by the space program and the promise of the Apollo mission. We eagerly awaited the first step on the moon with our extended family gathered around the small black and white console television in our grandparents' living room. At age fifteen, little did I realize the significance of the innovative technology required to keep the astronauts alive in the space capsule and on the moon. This technology launched a new era of innovation in medicine and anchored the trajectory for my future nursing career.

***

When I was four, I developed a persistent cough and had trouble breathing. My mom made chicken noodle soup and mustard plasters to loosen secretions. Common home remedies in the Fifties, plasters were made of dry mustard seed powder, mixed with warm water, smeared on a soft towel, and placed on my chest.

The mustard smell burned my nose and I shivered when the wet concoction cooled off. I didn't like them, but she said it would make me feel better.

I heard my mom talking to the doctor's office. She was worried because my temperature was 104; I remembered the number but didn't know what it meant. I slept a lot, and staying awake was difficult.

One day, I woke up in a hospital specially designed to care for children. I don't remember how I got there. I had pneumonia and was in a transparent plastic oxygen tent that covered the top half of the bed. My mom warned me not to put plastic near my face or I would suffocate. I fell back asleep, too tired to worry about the plastic tent.

Later that night, I woke up alone and unsure where I was. I started crying in my tent. A kind young woman in a white dress and white cap gave me a root beer popsicle, my favorite. I had a soft feeling of being safe and fell back asleep.

After a few days, I felt better and stayed awake longer. I curled my whole little body in my tent because it was calming. Another young nurse took me out of the tent, checked my temperature, and handed me pills to take. She bathed me in bed with warm, soft towels. She was kind, smiled, and made me feel secure.

"Your parents will be here soon to take you home," she said.

This was my first exposure to nurses, and it made a lasting impression on my choice of a career that would become my calling. I watched the nurses move with a sense of purpose, their quiet strength in the face of uncertainty shaping the image of what I would later understand genuine compassion looked like. From that moment, even as a young child I knew this was a path worth following.

***

Seattle was an upstart town less than a century old in the upper left corner of the country known for lumber, shipping, and Boeing airplanes. By the 1940s, the University of Washington (U.W.) meticulously assembled the Schools of Medicine and Nursing faculty, to transform the future landscape of healthcare.

When the U.W. School of Medicine (SOM) opened in 1946, it may have been difficult to predict its profound impact on the University, the Seattle area, the nation, and the world. The physician faculty's dedication, determination, and far-reaching genius formed a lasting foundation for the evolution of medical treatments. Determined to solve some of the thorniest problems facing the care of patients, *each* of these early physicians persevered despite being publicly derided with a *this will never work* public taunt at least once in their careers.

Growing up in Seattle, I took the remarkable medical care available for granted. I was born less than a decade after the Schools of Medicine and Nursing opened. My view of healthcare as a child was influenced by the innovations emerging from the U.W.. Healthcare in Seattle was unparalleled, and I assumed this level of care was available to everyone. We had the most current vaccines, safe surgical procedures for our tonsillectomies, and antibiotics to treat the pneumonia I got at age four. The Seattle Children's Hospital in Laurelhurst, where I was admitted, opened the year I was born. The University of Washington Hospital opened in 1959.

Polio was a disease that devastated young children in the 1950s and 1960s. I was only six in 1960, but I clearly remember one child, Tommy, in my first-grade class, was on crutches from polio. He couldn't run on the playground with us, and it took him longer to walk as we went to lunch or the library. He grimaced when he placed his crutch tips on the ground in front of him and used his upper body strength to scoot his legs in braces forward to meet the crutches with every step.

The polio epidemic became widespread before many vaccines, modern antibiotics, or ventilators were available to treat the disease. Children would spend months in a device called an *iron lung*, designed to help them breathe before ventilators were invented. A patient's whole body was placed in a large metal tube with only their head sticking out. It used negative pressure to stimulate breaths for patients with difficulty breathing.

The polio vaccine development and the successful mass vaccination program eradicated the disease in the U.S.. Mothers went door to door collecting donations for the March of Dimes, and we collected change at school to help pay for the vaccines. We lined up in our classrooms accepting our sugar cube with the vaccine sprinkled on it. Everyone was vaccinated, and we witnessed first-hand how vital the vaccine was because of Tommy's experience. The vaccine radically changed the survival rate for children of my generation. I learned to be grateful for medical miracles at an early age.

CHAPTER 1

Space Program Contributions to Medical Innovations

Tremendous technological progress was made possible by the U.S. federal government's unique increase in grant funding for research and development (R&D). In 1964, the money spent on R & D for the space program accounted for a historic high of 1.8% of the gross domestic product (GDP). That investment supplied the means to develop life support technology for astronauts in space. Only the federal government had the financial resources to support such experimentation. The results of that one-time investment in research gave us a precursor to the internet, developed by the Department of Defense (DOD), and lab and pharmaceutical research, funded by the National Institutes of Health (NIH). After the mid-1960s, funding and healthcare innovation slowed considerably. The average R&D budget for healthcare spending between 1929 and 2020 ranged from 0.0 to 0.7% of the GDP, far below the spike of funding invested in the space program. Throughout the 1960s, the National Aeronautics and Space Administration (NASA) contributed to significant advancements in medical technology on Earth. We underwent slower but steady progress in medicine in the last half-century.

In 1958, Spacelabs Healthcare, a medical equipment company based in Redmond, Washington, was instrumental in developing vital sign monitoring systems for NASA astronauts in space. The first space flight with astronauts James McDivitt and Edward White used Spacelab's technology during the 1965 Gemini IV mission. By1969, shortly after the successful Apollo 11 mission, Spacelabs introduced the first monitoring systems for the newly formed intensive care units in hospitals.[1] In Seattle, the proximity of Spacelabs contributed to rapid medical advancements of the 1970s. Spacelabs' equipment supplied hospitals with easy-to-use, intuitive, and accurate patient monitoring. As a new bedside nurse in 1975 I took all the data I had at my fingertips for granted. None of this was possible six years earlier.

The Seattle World's Fair opened on my eighth birthday in 1962, featuring space, science, and future themes. The Space Needle was built for the Fair, featuring a spaceship appearance with a rotating restaurant at the top. Boeing Aerospace was an active contributor to Seattle's image as a technological and scientific center due to innovations in aerospace arising from the Korean War. As an impressionable young child, I was excited by the depiction of the futuristic changes to our homes, transportation, and healthcare. I wanted to be part of this new world.

CHAPTER 2

The Nursing Profession Coming of Age

While the physicians in the SOM were developing innovations to help solve severe clinical problems, the School of Nursing (SON) was training nurses in the knowledge and skills needed for this new world of health care. Physicians and nurses traveled separate yet entwined paths toward innovation to provide increasingly complex patient care by nurses with specialized knowledge guided by expert physicians.

With this new focus on the sickest of patients, healthcare professionals viewed specialized care as offering hope for survival through inventions such as dialysis, central venous access, mechanical ventilation, cardiac monitoring, heart surgery, and bone marrow transplantation. Patient expectations also inspired the expanding knowledge level of nurses and physicians challenged by the new advances in patient care.

Nurse training before 1970 provided no exposure to the newly formed practice of intensive nursing care because those units did not exist. Experienced nurses began to feel exasperation and guilt over the number of patient deaths and their inability to supply safe nursing care with the rapid influx of innovative technology. This prompted them to find ways to learn the complexities of intensive care nursing. The design of the new units was modeled on the concept of recovery rooms developed in the 1920s to facilitate treatment for patients after complex operations. Nurses and hospitals were tasked with examining patient staffing levels because the specialized physiologic needs of those in intensive care required lower nurse-to-patient ratios than previously used. Intensive care patients were monitored, sometimes ventilated, and had central lines placed in their hearts to measure heart function and fluid status. These technologies needed significantly more nursing time for each patient. Such vigilance challenged nurses' ability to provide specialized, complex, and life-preserving care to large numbers of patients.

The long-held tradition of nurses relying solely on the attending physician's medical knowledge became unsafe because physicians only rounded once or twice a day. Even CPR was a physician-only procedure until 1965. Now it would be impossible to sustain that level of care. There were fewer physicians than nurses and the constant possibility of medically fragile patients with complex cardiac rhythms and electrolyte imbalances rapidly decompensating. The sheer volume of unstable patients made it impossible for physicians to be constantly available at the bedside, given the growing patient populations in intensive care units. The practice had to change. Nursing had to become more science based.

Frustrated about frequent patient deaths and their lack of depth of knowledge about caring for those patients, nurses organized to create pathways for learning about intensive care. These pathways initially began with nurses and physicians creating informal education sessions during which physicians taught nurses about pathophysiology, fluid and electrolyte balance, and cardiology. Nurses reciprocated by teaching physicians about bedside care and how patients responded to treatments. The difference between the high doctor-to-patient ratio and the lower nurse-to-patient ratio made the nurse's responsibilities to patients more complex. Nurses conducted more extensive observations and gathered physiologic data for the doctor who was spread thin across a greater number of patients.

In 1968, Norma Shepard, the director of the Cardiac Nursing Program at Baptist Hospital in Nashville, approached critical care nurses attending a physician-led symposium. She was creating an organization to support specialized nursing practice. Norma reached out to critical care nurses nationwide until she obtained enough support to create the American Association of Critical-Care Nurses (AACN) in 1969. The aim was to educate nurses about the increasingly diverse and complex units springing up in hospitals. AACN developed critical care nursing education and established practice standards to elevate future nurse preparation and clinical expertise.""[2]

Shared education and bedside practice created an unbreakable bond between nurses and physicians. Nurses' constant presence at the bedside and advanced training in intensive care gave them expertise and unique perspectives on their patients. I was fortunate to enter nursing in 1972, a few years after these systems were in place.

CHAPTER 3

Candy Striper

It was a foggy September morning in 1969, and a silvery mist obscured the top of the two-story totem pole, overshadowing Northwest Hospital's single-story entrance. It was a Pacific Northwest sacred symbol of welcome to the hospital community. I paused, soaking in the significance of the day. I came to this passion by way of my early childhood brush with pneumonia and the kind nurses at Seattle Children's Hospital. I wore my freshly ironed red and white striped pinafore (hence, the Candy Striper label), as my white tennis shoes softly squeaked across the pristine lobby floor. At eight am, the early Saturday morning quiet in the lobby belied the life on the wards. I walked by the vacant reception desk, entered the patient care areas, and followed the signs to 1 South, the medical-surgical ward. With sweaty palms and racing heart, I stepped into my first shift as a candy striper high school volunteer.

I slowed down as I passed the dimly lit patient rooms on my way to the nurses' station. I glanced through a few doorways. These are real people with real problems brought to life from my *Cherry Ames Student Nurse* novels. I hear the hum of healing as I reach the nurses' station, the quiet beep of a call light, ringing phones, clanking of metal charts returning to the rack, medicine drawers clicking closed on the cart, and nurses coordinating care. Everyone innately understood their tasks. How am *I* going to know what to do?

The bright lights of the nurses' station are a stark contrast to the rest of the ward. The nurses had been working since seven am and are well into planning their day. Mrs. Whitney, the nurse in charge of the ward for the shift, looks in my direction. "Are you our volunteer this morning?"

"Yes, my name is Phyllis. This is my first day." I offer, hoping for mercy.

"Welcome! I'm glad you're here. We can use your help." She smiles. "The breakfast trays arrived. You can deliver them to patients. Wash your hands before and after each patient, make sure they can wash their hands, and set them up in bed to eat. Let me show you."

She grabs a tray from the cart, and I follow her into the patient room. She greets the patient, introduces me, and raises the head of the bed using the crank at the foot. She then moves the bedside table into position and shows me how it works.

Mrs. Whitney was professional and compassionate. She looked like an angel in her starched white nurse uniform with matching white nylons and a nursing cap perched on her head. Nurses didn't wear pants and only wore scrubs in the operating room at the time. She was kind yet firm with the patients, knew how to make them feel better, and put their minds at ease. She was always busy yet never cross with anyone.

"Are you all right to pass the rest of the trays?"

I nod and follow her out of the room to retrieve another tray. Right then, I was hooked. I knew this sense of usefulness was a new beginning, no matter how small.

The greatest gift my mom gave me was to teach me to read at age four. As a pre-teen, I immersed myself in *Cherry Ames, Student Nurse* stories popular in the 1960s. I imagined myself as Cherry, living vicariously through a confident young woman who stood up for those in need, influenced their lives, and was a hero. For fifteen-year-old me, 1969 was a year of pivotal moments that shaped my career aspirations.

From reading *Cherry Ames*, I understood the rigor and expectations of nursing. Cherry exemplified the values of a nurse, which are foundational even today. She devoted herself to the service of others, became a lifelong learner, and was altruistic, with high integrity. Cherry was assertive and committed to doing the best for her patients. I embraced the idea that I could become independent and devoted to a career because of Cherry Ames.

My early days on the ward were mesmerizing. I learned a lot from observing the nurses as they went from room to room carrying out doctor's orders, assessing patients, comforting them, reassuring families, and working with hospital departments while keeping a kind and professional manner. I learned the values of the nursing profession from these extraordinary women.

The call to nursing crept into my heart right from the first day. I looked forward to my four-hour volunteer shifts, where I proudly wore that red and white striped pinafore uniform. Even as a candy striper, I belonged to a cause greater than myself. I found joy and a sense of purpose. I discovered the strength of conviction and the satisfaction of service to others. Through compassionate care to patients, I made a difference.

For the next four years, I worked alongside real registered nurses on a medical-surgical ward where patients recovered from surgery. I marveled at the nurses' confidence, caring, intellect, and control of the ward. Physicians briefly visited, but the nurses' watchful eye kept patients safe. They recognized when a patient was in physical or emotional distress and knew precisely how to help them. The nurses modeled a healing presence during a patient's most fearful hours. High-pressure and emotionally charged situations were managed with empathy, putting patients' needs above their own. I could tell the patients felt safe and cared for under the nurses' attentive gaze. I was captivated.

The more Mrs. Whitney knew me, the more she trusted me to help on the ward. I transported patients and picked up medications from the pharmacy. Before long, I discharged patients and took them to their cars, where their loved ones eagerly awaited their arrival.

In my brief time on the ward, the word *cancer* was whispered, a shameful taboo. Cancer was a death sentence, and available treatments were brutal on bodies. It would be another two years, 1971, before the National Cancer Act became law, another government investment in research would change the landscape of cancer care for decades.

"When you get done passing nourishments, please visit Mr. Lindgren," Mrs. Whitney said one day. "He's been feeling down because his family hasn't been visiting. He had surgery to remove a tumor from his lung, but he doesn't know he has cancer. His family knows, but we don't tell patients because we don't think they can handle it. So please don't tell him." Mrs. Whitney warned.

I tiptoed into Mr. Lindgren's room. I was used to having a newspaper or juice to break the awkwardness of greeting a patient. I explained my presence to break the ice with him. "Good morning, Mr. Lindgren. My name is Phyllis, and I'm a candy striper on the unit. If you have time, may I visit with you?"

Mr. Lindgren looked at me. He was an older man with light gray hair, green eyes, and pale skin, the color of the sheets. I could tell he had a lot of muscle at one time, but the skin on his arms sagged under the sleeves of his hospital gown. "Sure, sit down. Phyllis, is that right?"

"Yes, I'm a student at Ingraham High School. I started volunteering here a few months ago and I really like it." I fidgeted with my hands as I looked around for a place to sit. There were two chairs: a large, upholstered one stacked with linens for his morning care and a folding chair behind his bed that would require maneuvering behind him.

"I'm glad to meet you, Phyllis. The nurses here can teach you quite a lot. They're so kind to me, but they won't talk to me about my cancer."

Oh no! I held my breath. This was precisely what Mrs. Whitney warned me not to discuss with him. What if she finds out?

"Honey, I know I have cancer." Mr. Lindgren's voice was gruff but not mean. "They won't tell me, but I know it. When my family visits, I see tears in their eyes. I wish we could talk about it. I have things to say to them, but it's too hard for them now."

"What kind of things would you like to tell them?" I was curious, I'd never met anyone with cancer or who was going to die. I finally chose the oversized chair closer to him. I moved the linens to a counter. He continued talking as I pushed the chair closer to the bed.

"I want to talk about my life and share important things. I also want them to know how I would like my life to end, as much as I have a choice. I want them to know I'm at peace and accepting of my disease."

"I bet you have a lot of wonderful life experiences to share," I wasn't sure what to say. "What did you do for a living?"

"I worked in the shipyards. It was a hard job, but I enjoyed my years there. There was always something going on when the boats docked. We met sailors from all over the world. I assume the chemicals I was exposed to all those years gave me lung cancer. I know I don't have much longer to live. I can't breathe as well, and I can't walk as far. Even eating takes me so much longer because I choose whether to breathe or eat."

By this time, I'd pulled my chair closer to his bed because being farther away from him felt awkward when he was sharing such personal feelings. I kept thinking about Mrs. Whitney's admonition not to tell him his diagnosis. But *he* told *me*, so maybe it's different.

I took a deep breath and said, "What scares you the most, Mr. Lindgren?" I could tell he was nervous because he kept running his hands across the top of the bed sheet.

"It's silly for folks to think I don't know I have cancer because I can feel the change in my body. It's easier for them because they don't have to discuss it with me. But it puts up a barrier with my family when we can't be honest with each other. It's such a relief to talk to you about all this because there is no one else I can talk to. The nurses and the doctors kept saying the surgery was successful. I am not sure what that means. Did they take all the cancer out, or was it successful because I lived through it? I wish they would tell me.

"I worry about my family. I want to tell them I'm okay, I've lived a good life, and I'm ready for what's next. I want to tell them not to be afraid for me because I'm not afraid. But I know they're sad because they don't want me to go." There was a sudden dip in the mood of the room. Mr. Lindgren looked out the window. I didn't want to be intrusive, but he trusted me and needed somebody to talk to.

I took a deep breath. "What do you think would happen if you said to them, 'I know I have cancer?'" My palms were sweating.

"I'm not sure. They may deny it to spare my feelings, but I wish they would be relieved the weight was off their shoulders, and we could talk to each other about it." He was teary-eyed thinking about talking to his family. I reached over the side rail to touch his hand and he grabbed mine. His hand was cold. He'd lost so much weight I could feel his bones.

It was an extraordinary moment when this older man trusted me enough to talk about his end-of-life issues. I was young and inexperienced, so I spoke from my heart and desire to help him. That was the reason I was on the unit that day. I wanted to be a nurse since I bandaged my teddy bears as a little girl. Here I was, a young candy striper holding the hand of an older dying man, offering the best comfort I could.

Candy stripers also did projects to help the hospital and the community. We held bake sales to raise money for something the hospital needed, like furniture for the visitors' waiting room. During the holidays, we made large red felt Christmas stockings big enough to hold the newborn babies. They were discharged home in their Christmas stockings with their parents.

I took my turn being president and enjoyed planning projects for our little group. It was the beginning of my future leadership inclinations.

I was happiest working on the wards or with my candy striper friends. These moments of happiness compounded until they created days filled with joy. I related to patients, and my ability to alleviate even a small amount of suffering was a miracle. As a candy striper, I belonged to a cause greater than myself. I found joy and a sense of purpose when I made a difference in other people's lives. I belonged there at the hospital.

I obtained my work permit and driver's license when I was sixteen. I saved four hundred dollars in babysitting money to buy a 1962 Chrysler in mint condition. It belonged to an older widow's husband. I named the big, pea-green car Sherman, short for the Sherman tank it resembled. Once I had transportation, I worked eight-hour shifts every weekend as a tray girl in the kitchen of the local nursing home. In the summers, I worked as a nurse's aide in a nursing home, where I learned the basics of patient care, feeding, bathing, and dressing patients. Now, I just had to figure out how to be a nurse.

CHAPTER 4

Medic One

While I was busy volunteering at the hospital, my medical community developed one of the most innovative changes in health care. The Medic One emergency medical response system was a source of pride and reassurance for the King County community. In 1969, Dr. Leonard Cobb and Seattle Fire Chief Gordon Vickery created Medic One "one of the biggest lifesaving initiatives the U.S. has ever seen."[3] It is now the gold standard for emergency medical care in the U.S. and much of the world. Their method of providing prehospital care using paramedics—trained and supervised remotely by emergency department doctors—dramatically increased the survival rates of people suffering life-threatening conditions like heart attacks outside the hospital. This care was equitably provided regardless of ability to pay or color of their skin, a novel concept in 1970.

Before the Medic One program, people either died at home without care or were transported unmonitored (because monitors didn't exist outside the operating room) in an ambulance to the hospital. Most of the time, the only call made was to the mortician. This medical innovation felt like a true miracle.

The first Medic One call took place on March 7, 1970. That date was an important anchor and landmark in medical history, a turning point when we responded rapidly to patients with heart attacks and other critical illnesses. Dr. Cobb vigorously researched his idea about non-physicians performing resuscitation in cardiac arrest episodes. He was a target when his colleagues derided his innovative programs. "Everyone said, 'it couldn't be done,' and others said, 'it was a waste of time."'[4]

President Lyndon Johnson's Great Society programs of the 1960s created the insurance safety nets of Medicare in 1965 and Medicaid in 1966 which increased access to complex care in hospitals. A United States Public Health Services (USPHS) grant funded the Medic One mobile intensive care program. Thus began "a period of optimism, affluence, and expansion of medical technology after World War II and the Korean Conflict."[2]

As physicians and nurses were immersed in their life's passion of trying to address some of the most challenging medical issues facing humanity, the people of Seattle began to take note. A neighbor, family member, or church acquaintance had been given time on a dialysis machine, or the paramedics saved a loved one with the new Medic One program.

Seattle embraced the Medic One program as the stunning results of prehospital care emerged. These medical miracles didn't go unnoticed and began to serve as a source of pride. Before 1969, no standardized method of prehospital care existed in this small town with a population of about 300,000 people. Now, a new framework known as the 911 emergency system materialized. Our phone numbers changed from two letters and five numbers to all numeric characters to accommodate the new 911 phone system structure. Medic One's results were published in medical journals, and success stories in local newspapers inspired Seattle's citizenry and fostered the program's ongoing success.

The Medic One program was one of the USPHS grants the newly elected president, Richard Nixon, canceled in 1970 as a cost-cutting measure. It was on life support before it started. Dr. Cobb still needed $100,000 to make his vision of Medic One a reality.

When he sent a plea to the Seattle community in 1971 for financial help to save Medic One, he couldn't have imagined the response. The Rotary Club hosted fundraisers, the local American Heart Association contributed to the program's rescue, and high school track teams held twenty-four-hour marathons. Our high school enlisted my candy striper group to sell refreshments in a portable building close to the track as a fundraiser. The portable also served as a staging room for our high school's track marathon, where my brother and his track team took turns running laps.

Seattle citizens rewarded Dr. Cobb's original request of $100,000 to save Medic One by enthusiastically raising $200,000. Medic One funding was placed on the ballot in Seattle. The measure passed with overwhelming support, assuring the program's viability. Today, Medic One is funded by property owners paying twenty-four cents per thousand dollars of property value.

Dr. Cobb and his team used the funds to create the first mobile coronary care unit out of a large, rusty motor home, nicknamed Moby Pig. The motor home's conversion was done through intuition and inspiration since a mobile intensive care unit never existed.[4] The one and only Medic One was stationed at the county hospital, Harborview Medical Center (HMC). Partnering with the Seattle Fire Department (SFD) assured personnel trained in CPR rapidly reached victims throughout the city. Medic One's innovative approach to prehospital care was a layered response system using the nearest fire department. The precious four-minute window after an arrest to start CPR was essential while awaiting the arrival of Medic One.

Paramedics were trained in advanced prehospital care only after Washington State amended the law allowing non-physician paramedics. For the first nine months, physicians accompanied paramedics on calls to ensure the standing order protocols written by Dr. Cobb would be as effective as if physicians were staffing the unit.[5] Soon, paramedics communicated with physicians at the base hospital by phone or radio.[4] The Medic One mantra by Dr. Cobb was "to provide the quality of emergency care comparable to that of an appropriately trained physician on the site."[6]

The program became world famous because of the intense training of the paramedics. The out-of-hospital emergency cardiac care goal was a call-to-shock time of less than eight minutes.[7] Medics radioed short reports to emergency department physicians. The physicians then huddled with the charge nurse in the emergency department or the critical care unit to decide the best placement for the patient. In Seattle, Medic One patients were directly admitted to critical care, bypassing the emergency department. The system Dr. Cobb envisioned was now a reality.

In the first year of the Medic One program, sixty-one patients who were clinically dead were resuscitated and admitted to the hospital. Thirty-one were able to be discharged.[4] The average response time in the King County system was, and remains, three to four minutes.[8]

Seattle citizens also became willing participants in a massive research project guided by the research question: *Will Medic One alter the city's mortality?* The data showed a resounding *Yes*. Access to immediate CPR increased survival rates.

Medic Two was Fire Chief Gordon Vickery's idea to train the citizens of Seattle in CPR. A mere five years earlier, 1965, CPR was a physician-only procedure. Nurses or lay people could not perform the skill. Patients died waiting for a physician to perform CPR. Chief Vickery teamed up with Dr. Cobb and the Seattle Rotary. The SFD brought cardiopulmonary resuscitation to the average person. They started with the high schools.

"Everyone is going to learn CPR." Our high school principal announced over the loudspeakers one day. This was exactly the training I was looking for as an aspiring nurse. We learned how to help a heart attack victim survive if their heart stopped outside the hospital.

On the day of training, I stepped into the gym. Dozens of full-size mannequins were placed around the room. Each was named Annie and dressed in a navy-blue tracksuit. Next to each mannequin were alcohol swabs and bag masks to perform rescue breathing, another level of CPR for those trained in the skill. The SFD firefighters were teaching the class. They broke us into pairs and instructed us to perform chest compressions first, then rescue breathing. Once we had those skills down, we practiced systematically performing CPR.

We dropped to our knees as if we had just found Annie. We gently tapped her shoulders and yelled, "Annie, Annie, are you alright?" Then, the person finding Annie checked her pulse and breathing, made eye contact with their partner, and said, "Help, I need help! YOU! Call 911." The first person started chest compressions. The second student pretended to return, saying, "Help is on the way." That student then dropped to their knees and performed rescue breathing at one breath to every five chest compressions.

It was exhilarating. I hadn't done anything like that before, nor had I seen it done on television. I was among the first regular citizens in the world to learn CPR. In the first year, SFD trained 100,000 people, one-third of Seattle's population. By 2010, over three million people, an astounding 79% in Seattle, had CPR training.

A few years later, in 1979, Dr. Cobb and Dr. Mickey Eisenberg started the emergency medical technician program. Dr. Eisenberg also trained 911 dispatchers to supply CPR instructions over the phone to laypeople in 1982, thus enhancing the web of emergency medical services in Seattle.[9]

I was so proud. Now, I had a small taste of the meaning and practice of healthcare, even if it was just CPR. This experience cemented my decision to be a nurse. I put my heart and soul into making my goal come true. I started to take college preparatory courses. They all were challenging, but the most complex was chemistry. I struggled. My chemistry teacher lamented in frustration one day, "You'll never be a nurse. You can't seem to grasp the basics of chemistry."

My teacher's words paralyzed me. Suddenly, my future felt tenuous. He triggered my fears, doubts, and insecurities. I grew despondent that this one class would stop me from being a nurse. But I faced this fear of failure. I gathered my inner strength to tackle the problem. I studied days, nights, and weekends, trying to understand chemistry. I memorized everything I could to pass the course. Luckily, I had good enough grades in the rest of my courses, so the hard-fought chemistry *C* wouldn't hurt my chances of applying to nursing school. Math and science were important in nursing. I was curious to know if my teacher's comment was meant to motivate me, provide an accurate assessment of me, or just plain mean. I took it as being mean. It didn't inspire me, it frightened me. I remember his quote today and would love to tell him what I have accomplished.

As I approached my senior year, I started looking through the phone book for nursing schools to call them for information and applications. The invention of the internet was still two decades away. Being the first in my family to pursue higher education required incredible determination, especially in an era when campus resources and support were limited. Women's career choices were mostly limited to being a teacher, secretary, or nurse. I planned on attending a hospital-based nursing program like Cherry Ames, but hospital-based programs were closing while I was in high school. The American Nurses Association issued a position statement in 1965 urging education be moved to the college level. The education path I carefully constructed based on my role models, Cherry Ames and Mrs. Whitney, no longer existed. The historic 1972 shift in nursing education went from service-based hospital training to science-based curricula in colleges.[10] I applied for admission to the local community college and the U.W. when I graduated high school in June 1972. The community college accepted me. This was the first of many coincidences in my career during the most remarkable moments in modern medicine. I would figuratively ride the wave of changes in healthcare for the next fifty years. It would be the ride of a lifetime.

CHAPTER 5
Nursing School

The first day of nursing school in 1972 was overwhelming. The faculty, experienced women who were both helpful and firm, set a tone of professionalism and discipline that shaped our journey. "Nursing is a profoundly serious field of study, where people's lives are in your hands. You must strive to be the best nurses possible, as the well-being of your patients depends on it." I learned the values of nursing that first year; it was a respected profession with tremendous responsibility.

While some workplaces could take time in the morning to catch up with each other before they start their day, nursing begins at full speed. The minute our shift starts, we take a report about our patients from the nurse on the earlier shift. We must be alert and pay attention to what was done and what needs to be done for the patient. We already prepared paperwork about our patients' diagnoses and medications, so we knew how to care for them.

Mrs. Olsen, my first clinical instructor, checked in with me often as I worked closely with the nurse caring for my patient. Mrs. Olsen quizzed me, asking what my patient's primary problem was, what I was most worried about (*can I make it through this shift?...*

she meant about the patient), and how I could contribute to my patient's eventual discharge. I tried to have all the answers, but she asked tough questions.

"Your patient is on digoxin. What is their potassium level?" she asked. I blushed, quickly remembering she'd warned us in a lecture that we needed to know their level because they became toxic on the medication if the potassium level were too low or too high.

"I don't know." I sheepishly looked down.

"Well, you better look it up."

I always remembered a patient's potassium level when they were on digoxin for the rest of my career. Mrs. Olsen was my first mentor. She showed me the skills, knowledge, and attitudes that made a great nurse.

We rotated through many different areas of nursing to gain familiarity and to determine where we might like to practice when we graduate. We spent most of our time on the medical/surgical ward, reminiscent of my candy striper days. Critical care units only existed for three years, so we were prohibited in those areas.

We spent time in pediatrics. It was hard for me to see small, innocent children ill. The children with leukemia were bald with a few stray gray/blond hairs on their heads. They were so pale and weak, with large dark circles under their eyes. Early chemotherapy treatments were brutal on their tiny bodies. The survival rate was less than 20%. Drawing blood from their small veins was difficult and nerve-wracking. They were scared and crying. Sometimes, they had so many blood draws that their veins were hardened or collapsing, making the procedure even more traumatic for them. Loss of venous access meant they couldn't receive their life-saving medications. It broke my heart to hurt them, even if it were to make them better.

Pediatrics wasn't my calling.

Obstetrics was intense, bloody, and two lives were on the line with every encounter. A maternal death from an amniotic fluid embolus occurred during my obstetric rotation. It wasn't on my clinical day. The event seriously impacted the two students in the room at the time. They gave us graphic descriptions as if trying to process what they witnessed. Losing a mother as she was giving birth is one of the most tragic deaths.

Birthing babies wasn't for me either.

The scariest rotation was psychiatry. Trying to understand someone's psychological state was complex and disturbing for me. We went to a variety of settings. One location in downtown Seattle, Wintonia House, was an old hotel, repurposed as a halfway house for people with mental health issues. It wasn't a locked facility so the residents could come and go, but they had to return every night for their medications.

I was assigned to a young man in his early thirties named Jim. He was thin and unkempt, with long hair and a long beard. Jim's distant look in his eyes made me anxious to talk with him. I was twenty years old and this was unfamiliar territory.

I used a list of therapeutic phrases and conversation starters to help me. "Hi Jim, my name is Phyllis. I'm a student nurse. I want to spend some time with you. Is that all right?"

"Yes, my child, I can help you," he said.

I looked at him, not sure what he meant. I used one of my phrases. "You seem sad. Can you share what you're feeling?"

"I'm not sad; I have a lot of work to do here to help my flock." He eyed the other residents in the room.

"Tell me more."

"I am Jesus, and I can set you free. You are a sinner. I can save you from Hell." He leaned in toward me. He wasn't joking, his eyes now burrowing into mine. His appearance terrified me and his eerie voice frightened me. I did my best to keep a conversation with him and use my therapeutic phrases.

After half an hour, he was done talking to me. I was relieved. I found an empty stairwell to write up my notes for my assignment which took me another half-an-hour. I spent another hour in the stairwell, gathering my courage to go back out. My six-hour shift felt like an eternity.

I learned a lot at this facility. The people at Wintonia House were so challenged by their psychiatric disorders they qualified for Social

Security Disability Insurance (SSDI). They received their checks around the first of the month. Jim was missing the first week of one month.

I asked the staff about him. "Prostitutes hang out around our place when the checks arrive so they can entice the residents to spend their SSDI money on sex. There is nothing we can do to protect the residents because they have the right to leave the building." It was frustrating to watch this series of events unfold.

Even more devastating was when the federal government defunded and shut down community mental health centers, such as Wintonia House, within a year after my psychiatric rotation. There was no plan for alternative housing or psychiatric treatment for the residents who were abruptly homeless. It was a dramatic shift in public policy, one that immediately released large numbers of people with mental illness onto the street. Without a stable address, the residents lost their SSDI funds. It was the beginning of today's unhoused crisis.

Psychiatric nursing was out for me.

I was relieved to be back in the hospital. My surgical rotation started in the pre-operative area, to prepare patients for surgery. I was in the operating room and recovery room to learn how to monitor patients. In the operating room, I observed surgeries standing in a corner, out of the way of the staff. It was fascinating, but I spent so much time standing in surgical garb I started to get hot and dizzy. I worried about fainting. Once I leaned against the cold wall I felt better. I didn't get to talk with patients; they were either under or coming out of anesthesia.

Surgical nursing wasn't my first choice.

I started to worry nursing might not be a fit for me, but my next rotation was back in the medical ward. I felt completely at home there. I was now able to care for two patients at a time. My instructor this quarter, Mrs. Green, was encouraging. She continued to push me with more complex patients. I was *becoming* a nurse.

The graduation ceremony from nursing school was called Pinning, steeped in tradition going back to Florence Nightingale. We recited the Nightingale Pledge, where we vowed to care for all patients who are ill or need help. We also pledged to advance the health and well-being of the public. We each received a gold pin distinctive to our school signifying we were registered nurses. I was a novice nurse ready to tackle a new role. Little did I realize this ending was just the beginning. The actual tests of my love for nursing were yet to come.

Part II

Hospital Nursing

CHAPTER 6

Providence Hospital

Staff Nurse

I passed my state board exams in 1975 with scores reflecting my appreciation for nursing. Medical nursing was my highest score and psychiatric nursing was my lowest. Earning a registered nursing license was my ticket to enter the profession. A nursing license is a privilege, not a right, meaning our license may be revoked if we didn't uphold our professional responsibilities. Transgressions such as driving under the influence and drug diversion (stealing) resulted in our RN license suspension.

I landed a job in the tuberculosis and geriatric unit at Providence Hospital, a major medical center in Seattle. While I was in school hospital terminology changed from wards to units. My dream of being a nurse came true, and I had a front-row seat.

Soon after I started, I was charting at the nurses' station. Ruth, a seasoned nurse, interrupted what I was doing. "Phyllis, go check on the patient in 502." Her voice dripped with deviousness. Ruth's request seemed odd. That wasn't my assigned patient, but I sensed the duty to follow her order. I intuitively knew something was wrong.

In the brief time I was on the unit, Ruth grudgingly answered my questions, making it obvious I irritated her. I was optimistic, wanted to learn, and was her enemy. I happily responded to call lights and talked to patients and families.

Ruth rolled her eyes when I offered to help. “Don’t be so eager, you don’t even know what you’re doing yet. It makes more work for us.” She chastised me.

Melissa, the other nurse working, asked Ruth, “Are you sure you want her to go in there?” Melissa was kindhearted, in her mid-thirties, and typically happy. She was my ally and taught me a lot about being a nurse in the three months I’d been working on the unit.

Ruth snapped. “It’ll be good for her.”

I anxiously walked down the hall to the patient’s room. I arrived at room 502, tapped on the door, and announced in my cheerful voice. “Hello, Mr. Williams, this is Phyllis. I’m a nurse.”

When I pulled back the curtain, there was a fragile older man... dead. A large blood clot about six inches long poured out of his mouth. I was stunned and I panicked. I’d never seen a dead person before.

I didn’t know what to do. I looked around, trying to decide if I should pull the sheet over his head. Do I put the head of the bed down?

Shaken, I returned to the nurse's station and told Ruth, "He's dead and has a large clot coming out of his mouth."

She laughed. "Yes, I thought you should see it. Now, take care of the body and move it to the morgue."

"I've never done death care or seen a dead body before." I protested. I was upset and it was unreasonable to think I would know what to do with this situation after only three months of nursing. I imagined few twenty-one-year-olds had seen a dead body, much less one in his state.

Ruth tossed a box at me. "Here's the morgue kit. You'll figure it out."

I assumed that once I graduated from nursing school, my circumstances would be easier. I wouldn't feel so lost and I could find my way. My education prepared me for many situations, but a nurse who hated me was uncharted territory. How could she be so disrespectful to the deceased patient? How could she be so cruel to me? Nevertheless, now I had to care for the dead man. I told myself I eventually figured out Chemistry, I could find a solution to this problem too. I asked if there was a written death care procedure, hoping to find some clues.

Melissa shot Ruth a look of contempt. "I'll show you how to do death care."

Melissa was patient and explained the importance of respectfully caring for the body. She summoned the priest to give him the Last

Rites. We washed him and gently placed him in the body bag. We returned to the nurse's station to tell Ruth we were done.

"Call the orderly to take the body to the morgue." Ruth barked. "You need to go as a chaperone. There are incidents of orderlies sexually assaulting the bodies."

I was aghast. Again, my youth and naivete were apparent. I quickly looked at Melissa, who slowly nodded. I took a deep breath, called the orderly, and decided to trust myself to complete the rest of the task.

I helped the orderly transfer the body to the special gurney, which hid the dead person from any visitors in the halls as we went to the morgue. At the elevator, the orderly pushed the button. The doors opened and I nervously entered. There we were: the orderly, the dead body, and me. The orderly appeared okay, but I watched him out of the corner of my eye.

The morgue was in the basement, close to the delivery entrance so the mortuary personnel could remove the body out of sight of the public. It was frigid, with a stainless-steel table in the middle of the room. Cold storage lockers in rows of four-by-four doors lined one end of the room. We opened the door to a refrigerated unit, pulled out the drawer for the patient, and transferred him. We pushed the drawer back in and closed the door. I returned to the unit feeling like I had crossed a nursing threshold.

This was a graphic and traumatic first death, made better by Melissa and worse by Ruth. I later learned a term often used about this type of situation with Ruth and the treatment of new nurses. The phrase "nurses eat their young" was alive and well on the units. It referred to older nurses' horizontal bullying of new nurses because they still remembered how they were treated. It never occurred to those nurses to stop the cycle by being more like Melissa. Ruth tested my faith in nursing, but I had invested too much of my young life to give up so soon. This early trial helped me create a foundation of strength and resilience.

I didn't realize the culture clash in nursing because of the 1972 shift in nursing education. Practice was shifting so rapidly some nurses from hospital programs were leery of the college graduates. Some protested "this is the way we have always done it" when a different science-based practice emerged.

I lost my nursing innocence that day. I shifted from a wide-eyed, enthusiastic, and idealistic new nurse to one with a realistic view of the death, trauma, and fundamental issues of the profession. I learned to find my way out of a crisis and understood what it truly meant to stand by a patient's side. I persevered through trying circumstances. By doing so, I discovered I trusted my intuition. I promised myself I wouldn't become one of those nurses like Ruth, and I never was. Nursing is hard enough without bullying from colleagues.

We also cared for patients with tuberculosis. I learned a lot about respiratory isolation, reverse airflow rooms, and infection control. The remaining beds on the unit were for older patients near their life's end. Some had end-stage cancer.

At times, we also had older widows admitted for malnutrition. These women had been married for a long time, and their husbands preceded them in death. Most never worked outside the home. Because many of them were older when Social Security was signed into law, their husband's small amount of Social Security and pensions were all they had to cover expenses. Retirement saving options such as 401ks and IRAs hadn't been developed yet.

These widows were committed to their family homes and spent most of their precious financial resources trying to maintain them. Property taxes in Washington State increase each year, so they eventually ran out of money. They cut back their food budget little by little to pay the bills. I asked them what they ate at home and a typical response was they subsisted on reused tea bags and saltine crackers with cat food as their source of protein. Their plight haunts me to this day.

I didn't realize those early months were only the beginning. The true tests of my resilience – and the moments that would solidify my love for nursing – were yet to come.

CHAPTER 7

Certified Critical Care Nurse

When the unit I was working on closed, I was transferred to the Coronary Care Unit (CCU) and placed in a fast-paced six-week Coronary Care Course where I learned to care for critically ill patients and read cardiac monitors. This content wasn't covered in nursing school.

When I stepped into the CCU in late 1975 as a new nurse with only a few months of experience, direct admissions from Medic One were frequent. They accounted for more than half the patients. Taking a report on the phone about an incoming patient from Dr. Cobb was nerve-wracking personally. He expected perfection and attention to detail. I was in awe just being on the phone with him.

It was hard to fathom the changes in medical care since that first Medic One call in Seattle in 1970. Six years ago, few survivors would reach the hospital because out-of-hospital critical care didn't exist.

I learned everything I could about critical care. The gravity of my responsibility for seriously ill people caused me to develop grit when advocating for my patients. When someone died, I was terrified I had made a mistake, which led to sleepless days since I worked the night shift. I kept educating myself and became certified in critical care nursing through another rigorous six-week in-depth scientific course. Advanced education was a tremendous boost to my confidence. I did all I could for my patients; but they were in critical condition, which meant they had life-threatening and life-ending problems.

It was a heady time in healthcare. We saved more lives than we ever had before in the history of medicine but still couldn't save them all. Seattle doctors and nurses came so far in technological advances in such a fleeting period that the losses were especially hard when patients died. Bodies were worn out, the cancer too aggressive, or the trauma too extensive.

***

It was 2:30 in the morning when I leaned on the doorway to my patient's room in the Cardiovascular Intensive Care Unit (CICU), looking toward the nurse's station. I was assigned to the open-heart surgery unit for the shift. The lights in the unit were dimmed at night if everyone was stable. There was a peaceful quiet. I heard the *whoosh* of my patient's ventilator breathing for him twenty times a minute. He had several intravenous (IV) drips running on pumps that ticked like a grandfather clock. He was one of the sickest people in the hospital, having undergone open heart surgery two days ago.

When concerned about his patients, Dr. Lester Sauvage often slept on a gurney by the nurses' station in the middle of the unit to be available if something happened. I hadn't seen a physician do this before and I understood from the other nurses this behavior was uncommon among physicians.

Dr. Sauvage was well-respected and recognized for kindness to patients and nurses. He was a world-renowned cardiovascular surgeon for his innovative work in cardiac bypass surgery, performing the first successful experimental coronary artery graft (CABG) surgery in 1963 in Seattle. He designed artificial arteries and heart valves to improve patient outcomes.[11]

Dr. Sauvage was also known for taking on the most complicated cases some physicians avoided because those patients might die, which would reflect poorly on their patient outcome statistics. He took cases he believed he could help and gave people hope. He founded a research laboratory 1959 in Seattle known as the Hope Heart Institute, partially funded by comedian Bob Hope.

Nursing in the 1970s was patriarchal. When a physician entered the nurses' station, nurses stood and gave them our seats. We only sat when we charted. Most physicians were men and most nurses were women. If we disagreed about a medication or treatment, we weren't to directly question doctors about our patient's care. We found clever ways to ask questions to get the care our patients needed. But Dr. Sauvage wasn't like other physicians. We could talk to him.

When Dr. Sauvage woke, he sat his green-scrub-clad, tall, lanky body on the gurney's edge and rubbed his eyes. He caught me with all those reflections going through my mind and smiled. "A penny for your thoughts."

I shook my head to clear my mind. I blushed. I admired him. "Oh, nothing. I noticed how kind you are to stay close to your patients."

He smiled. "I want to make sure they make it through the night."

With that, he darted into a room. I turned back to my patient, marveling at Dr. Sauvage's humility and caring nature.

My colleagues and I respected Dr. Sauvage for his dedication to his patients. The nurses said he was devoted to his family and spent as much time with his wife and eight children as possible. His wife, Mary Ann, once said, "It was always an utter mystery to me how he worked twenty hours a day, seven days a week, would come home and be delightful."[12]

Dr. Sauvage was profoundly spiritual. He chose medicine over the priesthood early.[13] He focused on healing the whole person, not simply the disease. He respected each person's spiritual practices and thought it played a significant role in their healing. Dr. Sauvage believed in the power of prayer, noting it often worked better than tranquilizers. He earned the name "Saint Sauvage" because he gave over 5,000 Prayer of Saint Francis cards to patients and suggested they repeat the prayer daily. He was known to pray, "Not my skill but thine" during surgery to calm himself in tight situations.[14]

Dr. Sauvage's compassion touched my heart and shaped how I imagined medicine and nursing should be practiced. I watched compassion exceed indifference through his example. I was forming an opinion about what attributes made great physicians. He was near the top of my growing list.

***

"Let me show you how to mix a Dopamine drip." I reached for the IV bottle. It was 7:05 am on a Monday in 1976. A nervous first-year medical resident needed to elevate and stabilize a critically ill patient's dangerously low blood pressure with an infusion. I usually stood to give him my seat when he walked into the unit, but the power differential shifted that day.

Physicians ordered medications. Nurses and pharmacists mixed drugs and nurses were the final quality check before we administered them. Dopamine was just released from clinical trials and was a new drug for most providers. Even though I'd graduated nursing school only a year ago, my expertise was needed.

I showed the resident how to mix the drip because, as of 7:00 am, the nurses in Seattle walked out on strike. I took another half-hour because I couldn't leave my patient without knowing he had the life-saving Dopamine to keep him safe. The resident needed me to teach him how to mix and administer the drug.

It was six years since the first Medic One call. Nurse staffing patterns hadn't kept up with healthcare's breakneck progress from the medical research physicians and nurses conducted during that time. Before Medic One, half of all heart attack victims died within the first few days of the event, often at home. Patient care was infinitely more complex now than it was in 1970. Today, up to 90 percent of patients survive to leave the hospital.

Nurses became expert practitioners who used clinical reasoning to manage extraordinarily complex patients with markedly sophisticated technology. This changed how much time we needed to spend with each patient. Routine hourly tasks for complex patients included assessment, turning, ventilator care, suctioning, wound care, central line care, vital sign measurements, and fluid balance monitoring. More procedures took more time in addition to these tasks. If each task took 5 minutes (many took more time), then every patient encounter required at least 30 minutes each hour. If the patient or family needed comfort or information, it took longer. Or we might have a cardiac arrest which took more time and staff. The safe nursing care Mrs. Whitney provided in my candy striper days was in jeopardy. The starry-eyed candy striper was gone.

I was on the thirty-four-bed coronary care/step-down unit with one other registered nurse and two licensed practical nurses (LPNs). Patients in coronary care typically had severe life-threatening cardiac or respiratory issues such as heart attacks, chronic obstructive pulmonary disease, or pulmonary embolisms (blood clots). All were on the cardiac monitor, some on a ventilator, with intravenous medications (IV) flowing directly into their hearts to keep their cardiac rhythm regular and their blood pressure stable. IV pumps controlling infusions were a new addition to the unit that year. Before then, we used the second hand on our watches, counting IV drops from glass bottles containing powerful medications.

Harriet, the charge nurse, smoked, never mind the irony of the coronary care unit charge nurse smoking in front of the monitors. A short decade before, in 1964, the Surgeon General linked cigarette smoking and lung cancer. Almost 40% of the American public smoked then, twice today's prevalence. Smoking was banned in hospitals a few years later. Harriet ate chips and cookies all night to stay awake and only moved from her chair to take a break. She was middle-aged, obese, and mean. She barked orders and expected them to be followed.

Charting on thirty-four patients took a lot of time. We used paper charts and carried around pens with three colors of ink. The day shift charted in blue, the evening shift in green, and nights in red. No computers, they were yet to be invented.

The LPNs couldn't give IV medications, almost all the medications in critical care. Therefore, I administered all of them. All thirty-four patients were cared for by three of us. Harriet oversaw the floor and watched the monitors so cardiac arrhythmias could be detected.

A patient load of thirty-four made for very unsafe conditions for patients. The ratio of nurses to patients hadn't been adjusted in a decade. The ratio of seventeen patients per registered nurse in critical care, especially when one registered nurse never left her chair, made it thirty-four patients to one registered nurse who was a relatively new graduate (me), unsafe for patients and unsustainable for nursing staff. If I floated to the CICU, the ratio of patients with open heart surgery was much lower, with one to three patients per nurse.

My hospital's ratios were like other hospitals at the time. Unsafe patient assignments increases the risk of preventable problems, such as falls or infections, puts patients at risk for delayed treatments, missed care, or death. Unsafe assignments affect a nurse's practice and contribute to a higher risk of errors, injuries to nurses, burnout, and costly high turnover for the hospital.

Writing this description of night shift nursing in a coronary care unit in the mid-1970s makes my heart flutter. I experienced moral distress, a term that wouldn't be coined until much later in my career. It is when I knew the moral thing to do, provide safe care to my patients; yet I was caught between two competing and equally strong obligations. The hospital finance system versus the patient. I simply called it *The Great Tension*.

I was grateful to the LPNs. They taught me the practical aspects of nursing. The most influential was Liz, a young woman who called me *Honey*. She showed me how to take the most efficient physical care of so many critical patients. Liz, Susan, the other LPN, and I worked as a team to ensure patients were turned every two hours to prevent pneumonia and bedsores.

We started at one end of the unit, just making it back to the beginning of the patients by the two-hour mark. We skipped less critical tasks to make the two-hour goal. I took the more critical patients who required hourly care. The two LPNs turned the less critical patients alone. The most crucial rounding time was 6 am, our shifts were 11 pm to 7 am. Liz would remind me never to turn patients to their left side in the early morning. "Honey, it's too hard on their hearts. And the last thing you need at the end of your shift is for someone to die." She cautioned.

It was a Catholic hospital, and although I wasn't Catholic, I felt a sense of comfort in knowing the nuns and priests were available to patients and families. The nuns modeled nursing values of integrity, human dignity, and justice.

There were also traditions to remind us of life's momentous events. The loudspeaker played a few bars of a lullaby when a baby was born. When a Code 199 or Code Blue (meaning someone's heart or breathing stopped) was called, the sisters responded to say a quick prayer for the patient's recovery and to guide the healthcare providers' efforts.

That year, I discovered the significance of spirituality in the care of the critically ill. I'd been a nurse long enough to witness people die when they should have survived, while some survived when they should have died from their medical conditions. The magnitude of a divine being watching over patients gave me the strength to push through the physical and emotional demands of the work. I had always believed in a higher power and turned to religion as a young teen. The church's rituals provided solace. But this was a new depth of spirituality, of putting my faith into practice. I used my best gifts of thinking, communication, and compassion to ensure my thirty-four patients made it through my shift. It helped me work to the best of my ability when a patient's heart stopped until the house staff physicians arrived.

I treasured the nighttime view from the hospital's west-side patient rooms, with a sweeping view of Puget Sound and downtown Seattle. The twinkling lights of the buildings and the shipyards were a beautiful distraction. They gave me a brief mental respite to center myself from the seriously ill patients in my care. I performed my rounds carefully and, at times, anxiously when we had several unstable patients. I prayed before going into each room: *Please let them be alive.*

The strike ended when hospitals offered a pay raise so slight it took a year to recover financially after missing two months' wages.

We were assured rest and meal breaks would be mandated and respected. However, that has yet to materialize half-a-century later. Most nurses have eight-hour bladders because we don't have time to use the bathroom.

Patient safety justified 1,800 nurses walking the picket lines for sixty-five days during the first nurses' strike in Washington State history. We reasoned if we made the extraordinary step to strike, hospitals would consider the mounting evidence that patients die when there are not enough nurses. However, patient ratios were left out of the agreement. The Hospital Association wouldn't budge. They argued ratios didn't make a difference in patient outcomes. Nurses throughout the country continued the movement to address patient ratios, conducting extensive research studies demonstrating the relationship between patient deaths and nurse/patient ratios.

Decades later, copious amounts of data showed nurse education levels and nurse/patient ratios radically impact patient outcomes such as mortality. After thirty years, Washington State took up the discussion of patient ratios. As a result, the general *guideline* for staffing was one to two patients per nurse in critical care units and four to five patients per nurse on general floors, although this was often ignored in times of high census. The larger the patient load we carry, the less time we spend with each patient.

By 2023, medicine advanced even more dramatically. Patients admitted to general floors would have been in critical care in 1976.

Patients in critical care would have been dead back then because we didn't have the technology we have now.

Nurses strike not for a massive increase in salary, but a reduction in patient ratios for patient safety. This is the accurate measure of patient well-being in the hospital. There still needs to be national mandated staffing levels. California remains the only state with mandated ratios.

Imagine for a moment we replace brakes on cars for a living. On an average day, we can replace brakes on eight cars. But now more cars need brakes. Instead of hiring more technicians, each one must now replace brakes on twelve to sixteen cars per eight-hour day. Something must give, replacing half the old parts or skipping safety checks to ensure the brakes are correctly installed. This is done without your knowledge, and you are at risk of your brakes failing in critical situations. Also, how must the technicians feel knowing they are releasing cars with brakes that may fail? How long can they keep working with that guilt?

Now, add the complexity of human body systems in various stages of ill health and coordinating care among physicians, ancillary providers, patients, and families within a multifaceted healthcare system. Nurses *can* quantify our work similarly; however, hospitals often don't use that data to assign staffing levels. The excuse is nurses are expensive. If there were no nurses, why would a patient be admitted? Only nurses are at a patient's bedside twenty-four hours a day. Salaries are the cost of doing business for hospitals.

I returned to work at the hospital when the strike was over. Practice on the unit hadn't changed, except the few nurses who crossed the picket line were angry with those of us who stayed out on strike. The striking nurses wore a silver sequin glued to our badges to show we supported the strike.

The strike was my first reaction to *The Great Tension* between the constraints of fixed hospital resources for safe, quality patient care delicately balanced with nurse job satisfaction and burnout. To be realistic, hospitals have limited resources. Financial restrictions create the most struggle with quality patient care. Each side has equally strong, competing obligations: the system versus the patient. After the patient, *The Great Tension* affects nurses the most because we are on the front line at the bedside twenty-four hours a day.

Nurses are caught in the swirling vortex between hospital budgets and ever-shifting patient needs. At any given moment, a patient may need more care than the diagnosis on their chart indicates. Heaven help us if more than one of our patients becomes critical at the same time. This doesn't mean our other patients suddenly become *less* sick. Other nurses on duty may not be able to assist because they are experiencing the same dynamic with their patient load. We do constant bedside triage, resulting in moral distress and agonizing choices, leading to sleepless nights. Managing these two variables requires continual vigilance and creativity on the part of nurses and nursing leadership. We lead an incessantly variable human service provided within a fixed reimbursement system.

I spent the rest of my career dealing with the conflict between my professional responsibility for safe, quality patient care set against my job satisfaction and personal well-being, burnout lurking in the shadows. I navigated a myriad of significant ethical dilemmas related to *The Great Tension*.

After working in critical care, I quickly recognized that my associate degree in nursing left gaps in my education to reach an expert level at the bedside because some of the current technology hadn't been invented when I was in school. It was up to me to advance my knowledge and education to take the best care of my patients.

Seattle University offered an RN-BSN program where I took the remaining courses to fulfill my bachelor's degree obligations. I completed the liberal arts courses as well as the nursing courses about community health and leadership. One of the mandates for graduation at this Catholic university was completing a course in religion. I was worried it was a way to convert us to Catholicism, but a course titled *Comparative Religions* intrigued me, so I registered.

The course permanently altered my view of religion. The professor was engaging and creative in his presentation of the material. Speakers from various faiths spoke to us about their beliefs. They encouraged us to compare their religions with our own views. It expanded my worldview about spirituality. The common thread among the beliefs was a benevolent being followers embraced, who gave them comfort. The idea of a committee of compassionate beings from various religions safeguarding the world brought me peace.

I climbed the learning curve of a nurse and built a solid skill set as a bedside nurse, expanding my role in critical care. I was ready for a new adventure. When I worked at the downtown hospital, I was fascinated with critically ill patients on dialysis. The Northwest Kidney Center (NWKC) was a few blocks from Seattle University. I was intrigued by the dialysis process, so when a night shift position opened at the NWKC, I left the hospital. Nurses have a lot of career mobility, and I was curious about nursing outside the hospital's walls.

Part III

Nursing Beyond the Hospital

CHAPTER 8

Northwest Kidney Center

Dialysis Night Charge Nurse

Dr. Belding Scribner created the fledgling outpatient dialysis unit, the Seattle Artificial Kidney Center (SAKC), in the basement of the old Swedish Hospital nurses' quarters in 1962. SAKC was the world's first community-based rather than hospital-based treatment center.[15] Nurses ran the unit and performed the dialysis treatments.[16]

We had a plethora of innovations for kidney failure. Yet, we lacked the funding for equipment and personnel. Only three dialysis machines were available due to the prohibitive cost of the devices and the difficulty of the procedure. Dialysis is performed on each patient for four to six hours at a time, several days a week, thus limiting available dialysis machine slots. End Stage Renal Disease (ESRD) wasn't yet covered by SSDI.

In response to the scarce dialysis dilemma, the King County Medical Society President, Dr. James Haviland, proposed creating the Admissions and Policy Committee of the SAKC in 1962. It was also known by many names, such as *The Seattle Experience*, *The Life-or-Death Committee*, or *The God Squad*.[17,18]

Patients seeking dialysis were pre-screened by a committee of physicians and psychologists who evaluated whether the patient was medically and psychologically suited for dialysis.[19,20] Another committee of seven anonymous community members comprised of a lawyer, clergy, homemaker, banker, state official, and surgeon, reviewed medically cleared patient charts monthly to decide the patient's *social worth* to society. Criteria for social worth included age (under 54), sex, marital status, number of dependents, income, emotional stability, education, occupation, and potential contribution to society. Those judged most worthy were selected for time on the few dialysis machines, most often men supporting families.[18] Those not selected would die. This committee was foundational for the field of bioethics.[16]

Seattle was at the forefront of medical history as the community struggled with limited resources, rationing for dialysis, and the ethics surrounding the best use of those resources. The ethical principles of beneficence, justice, autonomy, and non-maleficence were in sharp focus as the committee's work evolved. Those early dialysis rationing decisions have implications for modern-day resource allocation.

Kidney failure patients wouldn't survive the two-year wait period for SSDI benefits to begin. Dr. Scribner dedicated his efforts to ensure SSDI benefits included ESRD without the wait period. He teamed up with Washington State Senators Henry Jackson and Warren Magnusson to convince Congress to pass the Medicare ESRD Program legislation to ensure immediate access to chronic renal dialysis for all Americans.[21,15] In 1973, ESRD became covered under SSDI without the two-year waiting period. It also allowed for funding to increase the number of dialysis machines in Seattle.

Once the procedure was covered under SSDI, dialysis access was widespread throughout the country.[17] The admission committee was no longer needed. Dr. Scribner's efforts to secure equal access to dialysis set the foundation for much of the later work on health inequalities.

One of the premier experts in bioethics, Albert Jonsen, Ph.D., professor of ethics at the U.W., was a vital member of those early discussions, which continue to this day. Dr. Jonsen served from 1974-1978 on the National Commission for the Protection of Human Subjects of Biomedical and Behavioral Research. He co-authored the pivotal Belmont Report in 1979, outlining ethical principles for research on humans.[22]

Professor Jonsen noted Seattle was an incubator for the field of bioethics, especially around the controversies involving organ transplantation and life-extending medical treatments such as dialysis. These technological innovations outpaced society's and the medical field's ability to fully understand the delicate ethical balance of using complex medical innovations to extend life *and* meet a patient's quality of life expectations.

***

Elaine was ready to be connected to the dialysis machine. Unfortunately, her Scribner shunt was clotted. Removing the clot was a physician's procedure, and Dr. Scribner was the patient's physician. It was 1977, four short years since dialysis had become widely available to the public. I was the charge nurse and called to let him know of the problem.

Little did I appreciate the national treasure we had with Dr. Scribner in the Seattle medical community. He was a humble man who lived in a houseboat by the U.W. and often kayaked to work. He arrived in his red beret and grey suit to greet his patient.

"Hi Elaine, it sounds like a clot is holding up your dialysis."

He turned to me. "Do you have the equipment I need?"

"Right here." I handed him the special kit with the sterile tools to perform the procedure.

"So, Elaine, are you still making that decadent lasagna?" He asked as he separated her shunt and deftly removed the clot. Elaine was well aware she would not have been a candidate for dialysis four years earlier before the SSDI funding took effect. She did not fit the criteria of supporting a family. She would have died of ESRD.

She giggled. “Yes, I use a new spice that gives it more flavor. I will make a pan for you.”

After a few moments, Dr. Scribner said, “There you go, Elaine. We can start your dialysis. I bet the new recipe is delicious.” With that, he washed up and started rounding on his other patients. That was it. Bedside conversations weren’t always profound, but they were a healing presence.

At some point in each person's life, their contributions and life's work might be questioned. Most of the physicians described in this book were told their ideas wouldn’t work, or worse, they were laughed at by their colleagues. Yet, their belief in their innovation was so strong they continued the work despite the doubters. The magic potion was perseverance.

Dr. Scribner was one of those remarkable people who persevered to create the team to make dialysis a reality. Nurses were the link between his vision and the patients. The medical community initially scoffed at his invention of the arteriovenous shunt. Dialysis was developed in the early 1960s to replace damaged kidney function. While the procedure successfully removed toxic waste from the blood, vascular access limited the number of times a patient could be dialyzed. The first approach involved inserting glass tubes into the patient's blood vessels in a procedure that destroyed the vessels for future use.[23] The patient eventually ran out of vascular access and died of kidney failure.

Dr. Scribner designed a Teflon loop, called the Scribner shunt, to connect the artery and vein outside the body. The shunt was separated for dialysis, the arterial side supplied access to the dialysis machine and the venous side allowed cleansed blood to return to the body. The shunt transformed kidney failure from a fatal disease to a chronic illness.

Today, patients are placed on dialysis using the same techniques Dr. Scribner developed until a permanent fistula can be created in the patient's arm. He attributed his success to his perseverance in problem-solving and his delight in tinkering with devices.[16]

Wayne Quinton, a medical design engineer at the U.W., created the U-shaped device. The arterial and venous sides of the Teflon tubing were held together between dialysis treatments by another invention, the Quinton T-connector. Both are still in use today.

Wayne founded Quinton Instruments in 1959. He pioneered various medical devices, from treadmills to cardiac diagnostic equipment. His motto guided him. "Never let lack of knowledge and resources keep you from doing something that needs to be done."[24]

The innovations kept on coming. Dr. Henry Tenckhoff, the father of chronic peritoneal dialysis, developed the first indwelling

Dacron peritoneal dialysis catheter and the peritoneal dialysis machine.[24]

Dr. Tenckhoff joined Dr. Scribner's team in 1964. Peritoneal dialysis involved inserting a Tenckhoff catheter into the abdomen. A solution was placed in the abdominal cavity, and the toxins in the person's body were infused into the solution by osmosis. The fluid then drained out of the abdominal cavity by gravity. The procedure was repeated many times over several hours of dialysis treatment. Patients with tenuous cardiovascular problems had difficulty tolerating the fluid shifts in hemodialysis, so peritoneal dialysis provided a more gradual and gentle treatment.

Dr. Tenckhoff's silicone catheter remained permanently in the abdomen. Before his invention, a catheter would be inserted for each round of dialysis. Tenckhoff catheters also develop fibrin clots, so when that happened, we called Dr. Tenckhoff. Even at the time of his death in 2017, his subcutaneous catheter was the industry standard for peritoneal dialysis.[25, 26]

Once the limited access to dialysis crisis was remedied, an issue later arose as for-profit dialysis units appeared. Controversy ensued about the wisdom of placing ESRD patients with a poor prognosis on dialysis to boost profit margins. Dr. Scribner expressed a moral concern over the business model, specifically the proliferation of for-profit dialysis centers. He noted financial rewards should not be associated with research interests. He weighed in on the controversies in 2002, forty years after the dialysis committee formed, noting three critical issues at the heart of the debate surrounding technical medical innovations: Who should receive treatment? When are science and technology used for financial gain? How much dialysis is enough?[20]

Dr. Scribner called upon the healthcare community to address the ethical issues related to the for-profit business model in the face of limited resources and the moral mandate to ensure the quality of life for patients.[20] The debate continues today: How much healthcare is enough? When are we prolonging suffering?

This exposure to complex ethical decision-making helped me grow as a professional nurse. I encountered situations where the best course of action conflicted with patient wishes, especially around end-of-life issues. I enjoyed caring for extraordinarily complex patients and found the ethical challenge of balancing patient autonomy with medical realities of life prolonging care fascinating.

I graduated from Seattle University, with my bachelor's degree in nursing. I was ready for a new adventure. A two-line advertisement in the *Seattle Times* Help Wanted section advertised "Pheresis nurse needed" with a phone number. I had to look up what pheresis meant. That tiny ad lead me to one of the most interesting jobs of my career.

CHAPTER 9

Fred Hutchinson Cancer Research Center

Pheresis Research Nurse

We were fortunate Dr. E. Donnall Thomas was the Director of the Clinical Research Division at Fred Hutchinson Cancer Research Center, affectionately called Fred Hutch. His early interest in leukemia during medical school focused on stimulating bone marrow production. At the time, bone marrow transplantation required total body irradiation to kill the diseased bone marrow. The bone marrow cells from a healthy tissue-type-matched donor were then infused into the patient. He conducted the first bone marrow transplant in 1956 with a patient's identical twin.[27] In 1963, he joined the faculty of the SOM at the U.W.

In 1979 the first Fred Hutch patient received bone marrow from an unrelated donor. This led to the creation of the national bone marrow registry. Initially, there were poor survival rates, but Dr. Thomas and his team persevered. He created a team of nurses and physicians focused on caring for children with advanced leukemia, aplastic anemia, or genetic diseases.[27] Dr. Thomas credited the long, cold winters in Seattle conducive for the extended discussions which advanced his work.[27,28]

It took one to two months for engraftment to take hold in the patient. During this precarious time the children lived in plastic bubbles, sophisticated environments sealed with complex air filtration systems to block germs. They took up half the room to give children freedom to move around.

I worked in the Pheresis unit on the seventh floor. We supported the patients with donated white cells and platelets harvested through *pheresis* until the graft was active. The pheresis process placed tissue-typed donors on a machine that took blood out of the donor's body and ran it through a centrifuge so the lighter platelets or white cells, were harvested off the top of the spinning blood. The platelets or white cells went into an infusion bag, and the rest of the blood was returned to the donor. The process took about two hours.

Patients and their families came from all over the world, having gained a place in one of the twenty-two precious beds in hopes of reaching remission. The Seattle community embraced the children with open arms. A dependable cadre of tissue-typed community volunteers donated blood components at a moment's notice to support the children's fragile bodies while they waited for the bone marrow transplant to take hold.

A new anti-nausea drug was introduced into a randomized clinical trial while I was at Fred Hutch. An ondansetron (Zofran) study compared this new drug's effectiveness with the current, older medication prochlorperazine (Compazine), which had many side effects. Within a month, the researchers requested permission to break the clinical trial on a *compassionate plea* basis. This meant the new drug was so effective that withholding it from the rest of the patients was inhumane. Ondansetron was a gift to cancer care, quickly relieving nausea and highly effective with few, if any, side effects.

Dr. Thomas's kind bedside manner and collegial approach to nursing and research staff endeared him in the hearts of his colleagues. When Dr. Thomas won the Nobel Prize in Medicine for Bone Marrow Transplantation in 1990, he wryly observed at his Nobel ceremony, "Everyone assumed this couldn't be done."[30] When he returned home, he invited the Fred Hutch staff to celebrate at a party with him. He donated the $350,000 Nobel Prize money to Fred Hutch.

There was enough research funding to supplement insurance payments to provide the highest quality of care the patients required. It was a reprieve from *The Great Tension* in the hospital. Bone marrow transplants were successful. The current five-year survival rate of 90% for children with leukemia is a vast improvement from 24% in 1970.[29] Truly a miracle.

***

Dr. Robert Hickman's indwelling catheter assured long-term venous access for leukemia patients. The Hickman catheter, designed in the early 1970s, provided vascular access for highly osmotic intravenous nutrition, which was hard on veins in the hands and arms. It was inserted into the heart for greater blood flow to decrease the danger of high-density fluids causing problems in peripheral veins. Dr. Hickman was originally part of Dr. Belding Scribner's team.[31]

Dr. Hickman's goal was to improve a patient's quality of life. He listened to the unit nurses early on, who requested a catheter to carry out essential access for critically ill patients without worrying about collapsed or worn-out veins. The children with leukemia I cared for during my pediatric rotation in nursing school would have a much different outcome today because of Dr. Hickman's invention. A Hickman line made the difference between life and death for these patients. He drolly observed, "They had to call the catheter something, so they named it after me because they didn't think it was going to work."[31]

Dr. Hickman practiced long beyond retirement age because he enjoyed working with patients. He was best known for his compassionate bedside manner filled with empathy, humility, and sense of humor. He was always kind and accessible to the nurses at the bedside. I'm grateful I was one of them.

Dr. Sherrill Slichter was the director of Puget Sound Blood Center and the Pheresis unit. She developed the methods for collecting and storing platelets.[32] She was known as one of the world's most knowledgeable platelet experts. She won a National Institutes of Health (NIH) grant in the 1970s to establish a national unrelated bone marrow donor registry.[33] Up to that point, only related donors were used.

Dr. Schlicter was also the Director of Platelet Transfusion at Bloodworks Northwest and a Professor of Medicine in the Division of Hematology at the U.W. SOM. Her focus on platelet transfusion research was vital to the recovery of bone marrow transplant patients. She developed the method to extend storage time for fragile platelets and explored ways to prevent patients from rejecting donor platelets.[34] She was the driving force behind making Bloodworks Northwest a research facility, one of only five blood centers in the country to hold the designation.[32] Dr. Thomas noted, “The bone marrow program wouldn’t have been possible without those techniques.”[32]

One spring day in 1983, Dr. Slichter summoned me and the other nurses from the Pheresis unit and the Blood Center. “A new blood-borne virus has been discovered. It’s rapidly spreading through some specific populations. People with hemophilia, of Haitian descent, and homosexual males are at considerable risk for this virus.” She solemnly explained the devastating news.

"Starting immediately, we're screening our community donors by asking them if they're in one of these three *H* (hemophiliac, Haitian, homosexual) groups. We can't ask which group, as this is an invasion of their privacy. We must ask them before donation because the Centers for Disease Control (CDC) issued a ban for blood products from those populations."

Fred Hutch, many of the major hospitals, and the blood center were all located on Pill Hill near the Capitol Hill area of Seattle, where many gay men lived. Being gay was spoken of in hushed tones because it was still disturbing to the general population in the early 1980s.

The virus was called the Human Immunodeficiency Virus (HIV), and the late stage of the infection was Acquired Immunodeficiency Syndrome (AIDS). The virus proliferated among the gay population in Seattle, around the country, and the world. It was always fatal and deaths spiraled among young men. It dramatically changed the face of the gay community in Seattle. The fear and denial associated with AIDS escalated the rejection of gay men. AIDS was characterized as "God's way of punishing homosexuals."

Tragic scenes played out in the Pheresis unit. Many gay community donors gladly came at a moment's notice to help a small child. Sadly, we asked them the screening question and watched the shock on their faces as they were heartbroken to find out they couldn't donate. Our question was sometimes the first they heard of the disease. There was a significant risk of HIV transmitted through their blood to the child. They were not only alarmed because they couldn't donate, but they were more worried about the child who urgently needed their platelets or white cells. The ban on blood donation from gay and bisexual men lasted forty years until the CDC lifted it in May 2023.

Entire neighborhoods, such as Capitol Hill in Seattle and West Hollywood in California, abruptly became small ghost towns as the death rate among gay men rose dramatically. As nurses, we stood by the bedside of the young gay men as they succumbed, often from AIDS-related pneumonia. They frequently faced death alone, except for the nurses and other providers standing by their bedside. We were there for their last breath, holding their hands since their families couldn't or wouldn't be with them. Uncertainty about how the disease spread pushed family members even farther away.

Still, life in the Pheresis unit went on with highs and lows. The highs were incredible when a child's bone marrow transplant was successful, and they could return home. The lows were overwhelming as we said goodbye to family members we had known for months, watching them return home alone because their child didn't survive the transplant. The work was all-consuming, and we strove to do our best for our families.

I learned many lessons as I worked with families whose young children were navigating complex procedures with the threat of dire outcomes. One of the most significant was the ability to read, discern, and empathize with the experiences of the sick child's family members. In the Pheresis unit we tried to make the experience of donating platelets and white cells as effortless as possible. We wanted a serene atmosphere where families disengaged, if even for two hours, from the harsh reality a few floors below. We provided compassionate care in emotionally charged situations, balancing our own emotions, teetering on the edge of compassion fatigue.

Most of the time, this atmosphere was a welcome relief. But when a child was clinging to life and depended on the platelets or white cells the family member was donating, that easy-going atmosphere might be interpreted as disrespectful and oblivious. This was why understanding a family member's expression was paramount.

On rare occasions, we received a call to immediately remove the family member from the machine and send them back to the unit because the child had died. Brittany was a four-year-old patient at Fred Hutch in 1982. She usually rode her trike around the unit, the nurses quickly following with her IV poles. She underwent a bone marrow transplant for acute lymphocytic leukemia (ALL). A month later, her platelets dropped below 25,000, a dangerously low level. She was confined to bed since she wouldn't have enough platelets to form a clot to stop bleeding from a fall, which might be deadly.

I was on Brittany's list of matched donors. Most of us working in the Pheresis unit were tissue-typed as potential donors for the children at a moment's notice. The closer the donor's tissue type matched the recipient, the less risk of rejection from graft vs. host disease. Children's families were also tissue-typed, including incredibly young siblings, who could serve as bone marrow and blood component donors for the child with leukemia. Parents or siblings were typically good candidates. Identical twins were perfect matches.

Brittany's father, Sean, was a match too. One day while he was donating, a call came from the unit downstairs. I hung up the phone and walked slowly toward her father.

"Sean, I'm taking you off the machine early," I clamped Brittany's dad's outflow line into the machine.

"She's gone, isn't she?" He searched my eyes for the truth.

I nodded. My eyes were so wet it was hard to focus on the machine. "I'm so sorry." I choked out. "She was so brave."

"Do we have enough platelets so another child can use them?" Sean fought back tears.

"We have enough. I'll make sure they're used." I quickly bandaged his arms and gave him a tearful hug before he hurried downstairs.

Her death changed me. The accumulation of children's deaths reshaped my approach to nursing and my entire outlook on life.

The burnout and mental exhaustion led to yet another pivot and job change. I was doing *the dance* of shifting practice settings when the mental exhaustion became overwhelming.

Part IV

Nurse Executive

CHAPTER 10

Snoqualmie Valley Hospital

Assistant Administrator; Director of Nursing

In 1983, I accepted a job as Critical Care Unit Manager for the new Snoqualmie Valley Hospital (SVH) an hour outside Seattle. A small, old district hospital served the area for decades but closed a few years ago. The community wanted a hospital for basic medical/surgical care and to serve as a critical care stabilization point to transport severe cases to the trauma center in Seattle, Harborview Medical Center (HMC). The new hospital had twenty-eight beds, two with windows looking into the nurses' station designated as critical care. There were four emergency room beds, one designated trauma/intensive care. The opening day ceremony was filled with community pride over this accomplishment.

The hospital was beautiful. Its location in the foothills of the Cascade Mountains was a stunning backdrop. The building perched on top of a hill and featured sweeping views of the valley filled with dark green evergreens. The lobby looked more like a ski lodge than a hospital, with a sizeable rock-faced fireplace and cozy living room furniture. The area was mostly forest and deer tripped the emergency doors as they wandered by the entrance the first year we were open. We wondered if they might walk through the doors, but they never did.

The position was a good fit for me. I had experience in large medical center critical care units and was a charge nurse at most places I worked. My work in the Pheresis unit was meaningful. But while more children were recovering from leukemia, the inevitable losses were taking a toll on me.

The census was low for many months until people got used to the idea the hospital existed. We recruited more physicians to staff the hospital and the emergency department to serve the growing community. Most of our patients in critical care were older people with uncomplicated heart disease who lived in the valley most of their lives.

As the critical care patients were recovering, they were often depressed, missing their home, loved ones, and pets. One Saturday, an older patient, Ted, made an unusual request. "I'm so lonely lying in this hospital bed and miss my dog, Heidi. Is there any way she can visit me?" He was near tears and was stable.

The doctors finished rounding for the day and administration was gone for the weekend. I whispered, "Yes, let's try it. But we must bring Heidi in through the window; she can't come through the front door."

He called his wife while I covered his bed with a sheet so Heidi could be with him. Soon, his wife walked around the side of the hospital to Ted's open window. She handed me Heidi and quickly came through the hospital's front door. I placed Heidi, a small ruby King Charles Cavalier, next to Ted and closed his door. I adjusted the blinds to the nurses' station to monitor him. He was on a cardiac monitor so I could observe his heart rate and rhythm.

The little family spent about an hour together before Heidi left through the window she entered. We were lucky the hospital was a single story. Ted's spirits lifted, he became more talkative and more receptive to our cardiac teaching. He went home a few days later. Soon after our escapade, research articles were published about the benefits of pet therapy. A decade later, most hospitals had dogs wearing hospital identification badges and making rounds to visit patients.

***

Many activities in our area brought patients to our door. The major highway connecting eastern with western Washington ran right by the hospital. Logging was a crucial industry in the area. We were less than half an hour from Snoqualmie Summit, the main ski area in Washington.

As the nearest facility to receive patients, we saw severe traumas. Ski injuries with orthopedic issues were common. Car accidents from the mountain pass brought an array of trauma. Logging accidents involved severed limbs, deep wounds from chainsaws, or trauma from falling giant century-old evergreen trees. The loggers were large, powerful men who barely fit the gurneys. They eclipsed my petite frame, yet they treated me with such respect, stoically saying, "Yes ma'am, no ma'am" to my questions despite terrific pain.

Most of the physicians staffing our emergency department were family practice who came from their offices during the day when we called them or spent the night in the hospital after their clinics closed. Emergency medicine was just emerging as a physician specialty.

Since we were not a designated trauma center, our purpose was to stabilize and transport. Traffic started getting heavier as Seattle grew, so ground transport from the hospital to downtown Seattle required long commutes for the medic unit to arrive at our hospital and then return to the trauma center at HMC. It exceeded two hours or more round trip, too much time with a critically ill or profusely bleeding patient.

Before the hospital opened in 1983, advancements in emergency medical care created a web of services for critically ill patients in our region. A new air mobile critical care unit, Airlift Northwest, was founded in 1982.[35] Founder Dr. Michael Copass dedicated his life to providing quality medical services for medically underserved populations in the greater Pacific Northwest. He was in Alaska when a house fire killed three children before they reached medical services. The incident deeply affected him, and he believed we should bring critical care to the patients. Airlift Northwest became the first critical care air ambulance service and now transports over 3,500 patients annually.[36]

Dr. Copass helped establish one of the top trauma centers in the world at HMC.[36] He was also instrumental in developing Medic One and emergency medical services in the 1970s. He was the paramedic training program's co-founder and medical director. He later added trauma care to the curriculum.[37]

Like many visionaries I was privileged to work with, Dr. Copass also received criticism from medical professionals around the country who refused to believe Medic One and Airlift successfully operated with nurses, paramedics, and emergency medical technicians.

I appreciated Dr. Copass's recognition of the value of nurses. He advised his medical students, "When one of them (nurses) asks you a rhetorical question— 'Do you think this person needs cervical traction?'—you'd better already have done it."[38]

Airlift Northwest featured helicopter and fixed-wing air ambulances with sophisticated capabilities, including advanced cardiac life support, neonatal resuscitation, and trauma care. Critical care nurses trained in the physics of pressure changes as the aircraft reached different altitudes staffed the aircraft. The program allowed advanced life support for the remote areas of the Washington, Wyoming, Alaska, Montana, and Idaho (WWAMI) region; the U.W. service area. HMC was the designated trauma center for the WWAMI region, covering about one-quarter of the U.S. land mass. Airlift was a vital link between rural hospitals like ours and the regional trauma center at HMC.[35]

At an altitude of 2500 feet, SVH was impacted by inclement weather. Mountain storms or low land fog at the base of the hill made transport a delicate balance amid weather conditions. Our hospital had a helipad in the lower parking lot. Helicopter staff were in radio communication with both hospital command units and the physicians. We stabilized patients in the emergency department, started the intravenous lines, provided respiratory or cardiac support as needed, and supported patient injuries. When a helicopter landed, we had the patient ready for transport.

Cindy was an Airlift Northwest nurse who frequently responded to our calls. One day, she arrived at SVH in her flight suit to retrieve a severely injured motorcycle accident patient. Another RN and a helicopter pilot accompanied her.

"We have a 38-year-old male whose motorcycle slipped on an ice patch coming over the pass." I reported quickly. "He fell, hit his helmeted head on the road, and the motorcycle landed on his left leg. We stabilized him on the backboard with a C collar. His left arm has a sixteen gauge IV with normal saline running. He's alert and oriented, and neuro checks are good. He has oxygen running at four liters by nasal cannula."

Cindy asked, "What has he had for pain?"

"A total of 8 mg of morphine IV."

"What do his x-rays show?"

"The spinal films are inconclusive. His left tibia is fractured in two places, and his left lung shows a partial pneumothorax. We don't have CT capability here." I explained.

"Okay, we'll get him to Harborview. I'll keep an eye on that lung. We may need to put in a Heimlich valve to decompress it in flight because of pressure changes. Let's get him on our gurney on three. One, two, three!" She commanded as my colleague and I each grabbed a corner of the backboard to scoot him onto the gurney.

"Thanks, Cindy," I said as she and the other RN removed him from our monitors and placed him on their monitoring system, which sat on a shelf hooked onto the stretcher over the patient. They hurried down the hall to the elevator and the waiting helicopter. I watched as the helicopter lifted off the helipad, waving to Cindy, who was now wearing a helmet with a microphone. I saw her reporting to the emergency department physician at Harborview. The patient would arrive in about fifteen minutes, saving precious time to protect his life. No matter how often we transported patients by Airlift, I was grateful and relieved that the patient survived this long, we could stabilize them, and we lived in a community with excellent medical resources not available in so many other areas in the country.

Airlift Northwest was the perfect fit for Cindy. Funny and bright, she was sharp, breathed adrenaline, and lived on caffeine. Skydiving was one of her favorite sports. She loved the autonomy of her job and lectured at local and national critical care conferences. She had graphic slides of all the traumas she treated.

Cindy continued with Airlift for the rest of her career, serving as a flight nurse and clinical educator for over twenty-five years. The American Association of Critical-Care Nurses featured her career life story in their 2022 Nursing Excellence series.

In 2001, Dr. Copass was rescued by Medic One, the service he helped found. He suffered a heart attack at home. Because of Dr. Copass's vision, Seattle was renowned as the best place in the world to have a heart attack due to the presence of Medic One and the high percentage of citizens trained in CPR. As medical professionals, we joked Seattle was the worst place to faint because, in the heat of the moment, some laypeople wouldn't stop to check if a pulse were present, one of the first steps in CPR. Fortunately, Dr. Copass had an uncomplicated course and returned home soon after his admission to HMC. I can't imagine being his admitting nurse. Not only would that nurse be caring for a physician with exacting standards, but he was also a national treasure.

***

In 1985, I was appointed the new Assistant Administrator and Director of Nursing. All clinical services in the hospital were under my authority. At thirty years old I had grown comfortable with leadership positions, since I'd been a charge nurse in critical care units of large medical centers with more beds than in our rural hospital.

Suddenly, my conversations shifted from the bedside to the boardroom. Shortly after I stepped into the role, the hospital was up for its first accreditation by the Joint Commission on Accreditation of Healthcare Organizations (JCAHO) to receive payments from Medicare patients. Since the hospital was new, we had to wait a couple of years until we had patient outcomes for them to evaluate.

I hadn't done an accreditation report before. Fortunately, a Catholic healthcare system had recently bought the facility from the hospital district. The community raised the money to build the hospital but defeated the bond levy to sustain it, so it had to be sold. The new healthcare system embraced our little hospital. Several more seasoned Directors of Nursing from other facilities in the system helped me prepare our accreditation documents from scratch. The accreditation visit went well. I learned so much from the experience, but the process told me I needed more education to continue at an executive level.

The sisters who ran the system were great at business. They repeatedly advised me, *no margin, no mission*, meaning we needed to be cautious with our budget. As the chief nurse executive, I was on the other side of *The Great Tension* and believed I would be in an advantageous position to balance fiscal responsibility, quality patient care, and nurse job satisfaction. However, a complex new case-mix system with fixed reimbursement for medical procedures, known as diagnosis-related group (DRGs) was instituted in 1983, the year we opened. The prior financial model was fee for service. Hospitals used to bill for care without limits. Finance officers said DRGs meant 'da revenue gone.'

Nursing is a team sport. At the center are the patient and family, followed by the nurses. Physicians write orders, but we have the education, skill, and context to deliver care. Patients may see their physician, physical, occupational, or speech therapist, and pharmacist as an outpatient. Patients needed the expertise of nurses who could assess, plan, implement, and evaluate their hospital course. We were the *only* provider at the bedside twenty-four hours a day.

This was a crucial point because hospital resources were (and are) divided between revenue centers and cost centers. Surgeons were revenue-generating because they brought patients to the hospital for surgery. However, when the patient left the operating room to go to the intensive care unit or general floor, they are cared for by specially trained nurses who are considered an expense (or cost center) to the hospital.

The strike a decade earlier inspired us to define our practice in measurable terms. Yet, nursing care is still charged in the hospital room rate along with housekeeping and dietary expenses. The argument was that we couldn't quantify our practice. We made tremendous strides in calculating hours per patient day and acuity to figure out how much nursing care patients needed. Because money is power in organizations, I argued with our chief financial officer and the Board that nursing earned a greater voice at the table in guiding patient care and resources. Our role provides twenty-four-hour-a-day continuous patient interaction, family support, and emotional resilience. It is the ONLY reason patients are admitted. The Board agreed that nursing was critical but *expensive*, so it remained a cost center. The argument continues today.

I could speak up for my patients. Now, I needed to find my voice as a leader. The weight of all aspects of patient care rested squarely on my shoulders. I compromised the safety of patients if I failed. I faltered many times but persisted until I remedied the situation.

I made tremendous strides as a leader as the hospital grew. While I had been a charge nurse in large medical centers, I had no formal education about executive roles. Tradition held that the best bedside nurses were chosen as the unit charge. We eventually discovered that solid bedside skills don't necessarily prepare us for higher levels of leadership. Formal education is required to manage organizational change and strategic decision-making.

I learned to be kind but firm as a leader. I didn't have to turn into a mean person. I could keep my empathy, which made me such a good nurse, while holding boundaries. Sister Mary, the health care corporation's president, mentored me. Through her example, I learned to be kind yet firm as a leader and use my voice to speak up for the voiceless with grace and humility.

Our nursing team volunteered in the community schools when off duty, teaching the Scrubby Bear handwashing program to the youngest children. We partnered with the local police department to present Nancy Reagan's national Drug Abuse Resistance Education (DARE) to keep kids off drugs program. The local public health department collaborated with us to teach high school teens about sexually transmitted diseases and pregnancy prevention.

I was invited as the first woman to join the local Rotary. I was honored to be invited yet on alert to participate in equal measure with the men, taking only my turn at administrative tasks such as recording the minutes. Some members thought minute taking would fit me well on a permanent basis, but I tactfully declined.

We opened without the authorization to offer obstetrical services; however, that didn't stop women in active labor from presenting to our ER, fearing they wouldn't make it forty-five minutes to the nearest hospital with obstetrical services. Eventually, there was a push to redesignate beds into a two-bed birthing center. The hospital was built with one surgical suite. If we added a birthing center, we had to add another surgical suite in case a mother required an emergency Cesarean section if a surgery was in progress.

Embarking on this modest remodel of the hospital required the completion of a Certificate of Need (CON) from the Washington State Hospital Commission. Once again, I found myself writing a large (two inches thick) document proving our case as to why we should be allowed to expand the hospital services. Hospitals must present all CON applications before the Commission in a public hearing. Nearby facilities could attend the hearing to contest the request, and the hospital about forty-five minutes away did so. The Administrator selected me to present our case to the Commission because I had the most clinical knowledge. I was over-prepared, yet I was still nervous. It was the first of many public testimonies in my career. Fortunately, the Commission approved our request.

After these two substantial projects, the JCAHO accreditation and the CON, I knew needed more education to be effective in my role. The U.W. offered a master's degree in nursing administration with a minor in business administration. It was just named the number one school of nursing in the nation in 1984. I was accepted as one of thirteen students in the cohort.

I attended school full-time while working full-time since I needed to support myself. The curriculum was grueling. One faculty member taught the entire program. Mrs. Wilson was a long-time nursing administrator at the U.W. Hospital until she retired to teach at the U.W. SON. She was a taskmaster with no patience for someone working full-time. Most students were on financial aid and scholarships, so they didn't need to work. I was the only one working as a nurse administrator.

One spring day, I tentatively approached Dr. Wilson for advice about a real-world problem. In the Pacific Northwest, spring rain and melting snow from the mountains cause rivers to flood low lying areas. Snoqualmie Valley was one of those flood zones. The hospital was designated as the evacuation center for flood ravaged residents due to its location on top of a hill. As the Assistant Administrator, I was tapped to be the spokesperson for the media. I took journalism in high school and was adept at reporting incidents, but suddenly I was *in* the incident. I turned to Dr. Wilson for advice. She was surprisingly kind in her reply. "Tie everything back to human experiences. People relate to stories." Her advice clicked with me and I still use stories today when I talk to the media.

Computers were emerging. Mrs. Wilson booked time for us in the university's central computer lab where the computer took up an entire room. We learned to send emails and create documents and later to run the data analysis for our theses.

My thesis was titled, *Resource Utilization of Nursing Services in Select Swing Bed Programs in Washington State.* As part of my duties as SVH, I was to implement a Medicare program called *Swing Beds*. Only rural hospitals could designate the skilled nursing beds to provide extended care for patients who no longer required acute care provided by the hospital. Once again, I prepared a vast document to apply to Medicare to designate two beds certified for payment.

The problem with Swing Beds in a small rural hospital was that patients would "swing" (change) to long-term care only on paper, in their charts. They were usually in the same bed, being cared for by the same nurses as when they were acutely ill. So, they believed the care they received should be the same as it was at the acute care level.

Payment for skilled nursing care in these beds was much lower than for acute care. The ultimate problem I addressed in my thesis was: *Do patients in swing beds use fewer nursing services than those in acute care?* The short answer was no. They received the same care, yet the hospital was paid less. Reduced payment might be acceptable for rural hospitals since a core group of nurses must be on duty even if the census is extremely low. At least there was some revenue coming into the hospital.

My nursing career advanced to the next level at SVH. Leading an entire hospital's clinical divisions was vastly different than being a charge nurse for a single shift of a single unit in the hospital. Even though we were a small hospital, we had the same departments and requirements as the large medical centers in Seattle. Systems thinking was the most helpful concept I learned that significantly impacted my leadership expertise. A change in one aspect of the hospital caused a ripple effect on the rest of the hospital.

Staffing was a challenge because specialty nurses were needed in OB, critical care, emergency, and the operating room. The census was low, averaging four to six patients per day so I could only afford to have two nurses on each shift. Two nurses are required for arrest resuscitations no matter how low the census dropped. I settled on keeping critical care and emergency skilled nurses in house twenty-four hours a day, with OB and operating room nurses on call as needed.

The Great Tension twisted on an axis at this little hospital. We were rarely filled with patients. Nurses want to care for patients so low census numbers led to boredom, not burnout. My new quest for nurse job satisfaction was tied to keeping them challenged and engaged while caring for fewer patients. Our volunteer community activities helped.

I led the hospital through three significant initiatives. I was no longer a nurse at the bedside caring for patients. I was a nurse executive caring for a hospital consisting of many different, interlocking systems, and complicated departments. The 24/7 responsibility for all patient care consumed much of my life.

Leadership positions were highly visible, so when I faltered, everyone was aware. Some offered support and advice. A few shook their heads as if to say, *how did she get this position?* The interesting thing about such leaps in learning was that sometimes my colleagues still remembered me as the thirty-year-old nurse who became the hospital's assistant administrator. Returning to school for my master's degree helped immensely. I now had a roadmap for decision making and leadership skills, and quite a bit of administration knowledge under my wing.

I was in that role for a few years and developed some strong opinions about how patient services should operate. In hindsight, I realize those beliefs made me successful because of my zealous beliefs about quality care. The downside of those views gave me blind spots and sometimes blocked my ability to hear others' opinions.

About a year after I completed my master's degree, I was interested in more challenges, and I missed working in a larger medical center. It was a defining moment for me. I moved the hospital forward and fewer challenges were on the horizon. I realized my career trajectory was marked by my ability to run toward instead of away from challenges. The difference in this perspective was a key motivator for me.

CHAPTER 11

University of Washington Medical Center

Staff Development Specialist

I was hired in 1988 as the Staff Development Specialist for Critical Care and Leadership Development, a new position at the University of Washington Medical Center (UWMC). I started fresh, with new energy and leadership skills, back where I was most comfortable, in critical care. I was now at the expert level of nursing, at the top of my game. I was a trusted resource for the critical care units and a mentor for the UWMC nursing leadership team.

***

Mrs. Kelley was a tall well-dressed woman in her mid-fifties. She stared at me with a tearful anguished look. It was 1989, and she was trying to be strong for her husband, staying by his bedside for hours each day. It was a challenging time since we'd admitted

Mr. Kelly a week ago. His health rapidly declined, and he quickly became a priority on the heart transplant list.

Transplant recipients undergo a range of emotions waiting for a donor organ because strict protocols determine how organs are assigned to patients. There were variable factors, such as how many heart transplant patients were awaiting organs in our area and how sick a patient was, which relentlessly shifted. Fewer patients were awaiting an organ, and Mr. Kelley's declining condition moved him up the transplant list, but a couple of times, a sicker patient received the organ he was hoping for, which was emotionally exhausting. Finally, it was his turn.

Now that Mr. Kelley was in transplant surgery, the gravity of his condition descended upon his wife. "Will my husband still love me with his new heart?" The regal woman searched my eyes for the truth.

Patients may have a personality change after a heart transplant for many reasons, such as the impact a life-threatening event has on one's outlook. Patients and families undergoing a heart transplant may have faced months or years of unpredictability surrounding the disease and the transplant waiting list process. The progression of their lives was suspended as they and their loved ones awaited a new heart.

Mrs. Kelley wasn't alone in her fear. It was a frequent concern expressed by heart transplant families. This was a life-defining surgery, the gift of life from a stranger who was clinically dead and kept alive on machines. The removal of their heart would cause them to die. Emotions ran high for patients, families, and nurses.

The heart is a fascinating organ with a symbolic emotional meaning. It is associated with love, attachment, emotions, and personality. It's why phrases such as, *he has a big heart*, are common. Even when we know most emotions arise out of our minds, when we say we love someone, we place our hands over our hearts, not our heads.

***

One afternoon, Dr. Richard Cummins caught me in the hallway of the medical center. He was a well-respected cardiologist and was the Course Medical Director for the Advanced Cardiac Life Support (ACLS) courses I coordinated at UWMC. Dr. Cummins also served as the Chair of the American Heart Association's (AHA) National ACLS Subcommittee and the National Emergency Cardiovascular Care Committee (ECC). Dr. Cummins led the development of the national ACLS guidelines, instructor manuals, provider manuals, handbooks, and textbooks. As emergency medical services advanced, he led evidence-based research on resuscitation, emergency cardiac care, and Emergency Medical Services (EMS).

Dr. Cummins was a staunch advocate for The Chain of Survival concept for cardiac arrest patient survival. The Chain of Survival depends upon 1) early CPR, 2) early defibrillation, and 3) early advanced care.[40] He was an early adopter of the Automatic External Defibrillator (AED).[41] By 1994, an editorial in the *New York Times* offered "Why So Many Die Needlessly: Broken Rescue Chain."[42] While the Seattle experience was successful, with survival rates for cardiac arrest victims of 1 in 5, the rest of the country was lagging in such impressive outcomes. In New York City, only 1 in 100 people survived an out-of-hospital cardiac arrest due to traffic congestion.

Dr. Cummins weighed in on the issue by noting that 70 percent of cardiac arrests occur at home. Families of patients at substantial risk for cardiac arrest should consider purchasing a home AED for $1,000-$4,000 *and* learn how to use it. This was particularly important in New York City, where EMS response times averaged 11.4 minutes, dangerously close to the 10–15-minute standard window advised after the onset of cardiac arrest. In 2005, Dr. Cummins was given the Giants of CPR Award for his landmark contributions to emergency medical services.

Now, he leaned against the hallway wall and asked, "Would you be interested in being the Beta test site for the new ACLS guidelines?"

We had a good working relationship, so I said, "Sure, what does it entail?"

He continued, "The National ACLS Subcommittee of the AHA has redesigned ACLS courses so they're more student-focused and less punitive. The subcommittee updated the materials to reflect the current research, and we also want to implement this fresh style of teaching the course."

"Sounds exciting. Let's do it!" I said.

ACLS was developed by the AHA in 1974, four years after the first Medic One call. ACLS protocols serve as standing orders for nurses in the hospital and paramedics in the field to provide lifesaving medications and procedures without a physician during an arrest. The protocols were updated in 1980 and 1986. It was now 1992. Before this time, ACLS was nerve-racking. There was tremendous pressure on course attendees to perfect their advanced skills. Attendees had a couple of practice sessions and then were called into the testing room to demonstrate their skills. The discussion at the AHA was whether this type of stressful teaching environment promoted long-term recall of the material. The focus on individual performance wasn't conducive to fostering effective teamwork.

Dr. Cummins planned to teach the next ACLS course with the proposed 1992 guidelines, which focused on teamwork, mastering skills, and remediation for those who were unsuccessful in showing ability. He wished to promote the concept of Chain of Survival.

We decided course participants would include critical care nurses and resident physicians in teams to practice and perform final skill demonstrations. The teams then debriefed with the station instructor, focusing on what went well and how their performance could be improved.

I was a critical care nurse certified in Basic Life Support (BLS) and Advanced Cardiac Life Support (ACLS). I was also a certified BLS and ACLS instructor. I participated in various fundraisers for the AHA and was immersed in cardiac care. The ability to work side by side with Dr. Cummins was a joy and privilege. He was open, dedicated, and passionate about educating nurse and physician teams on the latest emergency cardiac care research. To this day, I learned the most about ACLS from this Beta test course with Dr. Cummins as the Course Director.

By this point in my career, I hit my stride as an experienced leader and expert clinician. I had adequate resources to complete my teaching duties and temporarily sidestepped *The Great Tension*. I made an impact in Seattle but was restless for new experiences.

Part V

Non-Profit Association Nursing

CHAPTER 12

American Association of Critical-Care Nurses

Education Specialist

While working at UWMC, I held a two-year term volunteering for the AACN National Education Committee. In early 1993, I spent a weekend attending the committee meeting in Baltimore. I shared a cab back to the airport with Fran, the Program Development Director. She was bright, intelligent, funny, and direct. "I have an Education Specialist position available at the national office. It would be a great fit for you. Have you ever considered leaving Seattle?"

I was astounded. "What does the position entail? Must I move to California?"

"It's a paid staff position in Aliso Viejo in Southern California." She explained. "All staff positions work in the national office. It's a dynamic place with lots of energy. The Program Development Specialist is responsible for coordinating the educational programming for National Teaching Institute (NTI)."

My eyes widened as I turned in my seat and leaned in. "I never imagined working there. I pictured it as some think tank with geniuses."

"It is." She giggled. "Crazy ones at that. It's the ride of a lifetime."

I was teaching critical care nursing and leadership development at UWMC and was active in the local chapter of AACN. I loved Seattle and had never considered leaving the city. I pondered her request.

My career was established here, but I'd been at the university for four years. I enjoyed the beauty of Washington, except it rained a lot, and we were talking Southern California with sunshine and beaches!

This was an opportunity of a lifetime that I couldn't resist. I admired AACN as an association. It's the world's largest specialty nursing organization, with over 75,000 members. This is the same organization that Norma Shepard created in 1969. It's mission was to educate nurses about the progressively more diverse and complex units springing up in hospitals.[2]

AACN set critical care standards, advanced research, and advocated for nurses, patients, and families. The patient and family focus appealed to me because we don't just treat patients, their families are involved as well but are often ignored. AACN also hosted one of the largest nursing conferences in the world, the NTI. Over 7,500 nurses attended every year, with 2,000 exhibitors. Only a few cities in the country were large enough to host the event, as it took over entire convention centers and most of the city's hotel space. The general session room took up two exhibit halls. The exhibit showcase accompanying the education sessions took up the equivalent of three football fields.

I attended the conference once in San Francisco. It was an incredible learning experience with so much to digest. The opening session was packed with critical care nurses. Famous people were keynote speakers, such as Congresswoman Patricia Schroeder and actor Ben Vereen, who expressed gratitude to the critical care nurses who cared for him after his stroke. The motivational speakers filled me with pride and renewed my commitment to my practice. Critical care nursing was intense and required every ounce of my mental, physical, and emotional energy to complete each shift. The NTI harnessed all that power and inspired nurses to continue.

I was both intrigued and conflicted. This was my chance to influence *The Great Tension* from a national policy level. I would later reflect back on this moment when AACN conducted research in the 1990s to validate optimal staffing levels and the impact ratios had on patient outcomes. AACN advocated for specific nurse-to-patient ratios based on those research findings. It wasn't until January 1, 2004, that California became the first and still the only state to legislate minimum RN-to-patient ratios by law. A nurse-to-patient ratio of 1:2 was established for non-ventilated critical care patients. Ratios of 1:1 were set for trauma patients or those on a ventilator.

The 1:34 ratio I experienced as a new nurse in critical care would no longer be permitted, a powerful example of how dramatically nursing standards had evolved. Today, that ratio would be deemed unsafe, a striking illustration of the importance of advocating for safe patient care and reasonable workloads to ease *The Great Tension*.

AACN made significant contributions to bedside practice. It was this type of advocacy that appealed to me. What a fantastic career opportunity but what a significant personal cost. I flew to Aliso Viejo for an interview. It took an entire day.

Sarah Sanford, the organization's Chief Executive Officer (CEO), was from our local chapter in Seattle. Her career started as a critical care nurse in several Seattle hospitals. As her leadership skills grew, the Seattle healthcare community recognized her leadership acumen. She became the Senior Vice President of Patient Care at Overlake Hospital. Sarah contributed her expertise on the national stage, serving on the AACN Board of Directors and as President of the organization a few years before she became CEO.

Her work advancing quality care for critically ill patients and families made her well-suited to lead AACN. Among her many enduring contributions were publications such as the *Standards of Nursing Care of the Critically Ill* and *The AACN Synergy Model for Clinical Excellence*. She was instrumental in initiatives such as the AACN Certification Corporation, Innovision Communications, and revitalized the Foundation for Critical

Care by bringing it under the AACN umbrella. She envisioned effective nursing practice as part of an interdisciplinary team. She forged strong partnerships with physician and healthcare organizations.

Any of these contributions would be a worthy lifetime accomplishment. Sarah's unique vision is as significant today as it was three decades ago. She recognized the rapid changes in healthcare and sought to remain relevant and at the forefront of critical care. Sarah's contributions to healthcare earned her induction as a Fellow in the American Academy of Nurses (FAAN), a prestigious honor recognizing exceptional accomplishments in nursing.

Sarah was vibrant. When she entered the room, an energy permeated the air. She was intelligent, quick, sharp, and expected the best from her team. I never met anyone with such a dynamic presence. Well-dressed and self-assured, she leaned into a conversation and made piercing eye contact.

My first meeting with her was in her office, which had a sweeping view of Aliso Viejo and the Saddleback Mountains. There were elegant paintings of horses on the walls and graceful horse statues on the tables in her office. I knew of her; she didn't know me. She welcomed me. "Professional development has long been an interest of mine. At AACN, we help members be successful in their profession. This is a fundamental factor for our mission. I hope you will enjoy it here. I'm from Seattle as well. The weather here is delightful, but it takes a while to get used to the more subtle change in seasons than Seattle's."

Fran met me after our meeting. "Sarah brings immense passion to everything she does. She won't accept a challenge unless she truly believes in it."

Sarah's vision launched AACN into unparalleled opportunities. The prospect of working for her was enticing. Over one hundred people were employed at the national office, and the energy was magnetic. Only a few nurses worked there. They were supported by creative and skilled professionals in information technology, advocacy, education, research, customer service, and public relations. Fran was right; this was the chance of a lifetime.

Leaving the medical center was difficult because I enjoyed the work, and leaving my friends was heartbreaking. Some UWMC critical care nurses threw me a farewell party at the *Pink Door* restaurant in the Pike Place Market. We wore prom dresses and rented a limousine. For fun, they bought me a palm reading with a woman in a corner of the restaurant. The woman examined my palm and said many things, but I left with this observation:

"You are undertaking a major life change. It's as if you are jumping off a cliff."

"How does it turn out?" I asked.

"I can't tell you." She smiled.

I thought *great, she won either way*, but it captured how I felt about the move.

***

A dear friend drove down with me to California. I cried until we reached Portland, uncertain about letting go of my support system in Seattle without one in California. The NTI was in Anaheim a week after I arrived. I stayed in a hotel, homesick and unsettled, until my apartment was ready. There were so many endings, and I couldn't grasp the beginnings yet.

Attending the NTI was awe-inspiring. *Working* the NTI was overwhelming. We were on-site for seven days for the five-day conference, creating the elements to make the event unique. It was particularly magical because we were in Anaheim. There was a private party on Wednesday evening. Disneyland was closed to everyone but the NTI attendees, speakers, staff, and exhibitors.

As staff, we worked twelve-to-sixteen-hour days, but they flew by with so many activities, meetings, and events that could only happen in this venue. We were an international organization with chapters in many countries. We met with our counterparts from all over the world when they attended the meeting.

I was so exhausted by Wednesday I seriously reconsidered whether I should go to Disneyland. Rachel, the meeting services director, recommended I go. "All the exhaustion we feel is relieved with the thrill of those Wednesday evening parties," she said. "It's where we can relax and enjoy ourselves, the attendees, speakers, and exhibitors."

Since the 10,000 of us had the run of Disneyland, there were few lines. I met up with my Seattle friends who attended. We rode the Pirates of the Caribbean, then ran to the Haunted Mansion. We kept it up all night, finally singing our way through *It's a Small World.*

Rachel was right. As hard as we worked, we used the event to celebrate our profession and colleagues in a powerful way. It was exhilarating and gave me the energy to make the last day on Thursday a meaningful end to the conference.

Monday arrived, my first actual day in the office not dedicated to making the NTI possible. I collated and synthesized the evaluations from the 7,500 NTI participants. I was to report the findings at our all-team NTI wrap-up meeting.

The comments were positive, some constructive, and a few hilarious. Wanting to make my report more engaging, I made a list of the funny and positive comments. I typed them in a lengthy list and cut them into small strips. I sent the strips to a fortune cookie company in Seattle to make fortune cookies with a comment inserted in each one.

The team loved it. They cracked open their cookies and shouted out the comments.

"Loved Opening Session, the President was so inspirational!"

"Disneyland was a blast."

"My favorite exhibit was where we could practice patient simulated scenarios."

"So many sessions. Next time, I need to bring my team to cover all of them."

"The 12 Lead EKG session was the best!"

"I filled a suitcase with giveaways from the exhibitors for the team at home."

The fortune cookie experiment succeeded, putting a spring in our step as we planned the next NTI in Atlanta. A task force of expert critical care nurses from across the country met over an extended weekend in Anaheim to plan the program. The task force members reviewed mounds of proposals kept in bankers' boxes, which lined an entire wall in the hotel meeting room. Experts in pediatrics, neonates, coronary care, trauma, intensive care, advanced practice, burns, leadership, research, and other specialties reviewed the proposals submitted by educators across the country and the world.

The experts proposed the sessions they believed were innovative and a compelling session for the conference. The neonatal specialist read a proposal, "This session on ECMO (Extracorporeal Membrane Oxygenation) is innovative for our neonates and something we need to offer. The speaker is proficient working with the technology in a major medical center."

We accepted the ECMO session. Hundreds of sessions were offered in the five-day conference, all selected by this expert group of volunteers. The task force chair and I facilitated the planning meetings.

The meeting was as intense as the conference, with long days reviewing proposals. Yet, the evenings were made special for the volunteers when we hosted them for a dinner or outing somewhere unique. I recognized Fran was right; this was the experience of a lifetime, and I was fortunate enough to have a seat at the table.

It was in California that I understood my unique experience in Seattle. Working alongside Drs. Scribner, Hickman, and Cummins was a transformative experience, especially given the widespread impact of their innovations. They didn't practice in California yet their inventions were widely used. That realization was when I understood the rare opportunity I had to learn from these great physicians in Seattle.

Back at the office, my work at AACN was all-consuming, with more than a forty-hour work week. I traveled to the East Coast several times a month and often worked twenty days in a row. It was tiring but inspiring work.

I had other duties in addition to the educational programming for the NTI. One of the first initiatives I brought to the organization was the standardized critical care orientation program we created at the Puget Sound Chapter of AACN. Seattle had thirteen hospitals, and the critical care educators from each hospital joined together to develop and teach a standardized critical care orientation course for many years. It was pure genius on the part of the educators who started the program. I joined as the curriculum was being updated and revised. Instead of thirteen educators teaching cardiac arrhythmias in each hospital, we pulled the orientees from all the hospitals into one session room. The educators took turns teaching their specialty. The orientees learned from diverse educators and the efficient teaching freed up time for us to tackle other much-needed projects in our hospitals.

My friend Cindy, from Airlift Northwest, was one of the instructors. Her favorite case was a head trauma with an axe lodged in someone's head. Her favorite question to students was, "Do you remove the axe?" (The answer is no.) She told students she "cares for patients on the worst day of their life."[39]

I received many calls at AACN from smaller hospitals around the country asking for orientation materials to help them educate their new nurses. We had a variety of excellent materials but not one curriculum that could be an instant, state-of-the-art course for these educators. I contacted the Puget Sound Chapter president and asked her to be the editor for a curriculum we adapted for national audiences. She was excited for the opportunity and engaged all the critical care educators in the Seattle consortium to serve as authors. We created notebooks for educators, including instructor manuals with lecture outlines, supporting materials, and overhead projector slides. We also created a notebook with master copies of lecture outlines to be copied for the participants. We spent a great deal of effort producing the paper materials.

The Essentials of Critical Care Orientation (ECCO) program became an instant success nationwide, with many hospitals purchasing the program. At the same time, the Internet started to debut to the average American. Our education resource specialist, who wasn't a nurse but was creative in the new field of electronic media, started to prepare the ECCO program's online version.

Director of Professional Development

The Internet opened a whole new world for educational resources. One day, as the new Director of Professional Development, I received a call from a new start-up company called WebMD. They were interested in hosting our educational materials on their website. They offered to bring me and some education team members to Atlanta to make their pitch. I agreed, and our team flew to meet this new company in a small office in a strip mall. Their team was intelligent and animated about the future and what the Internet could do for medicine and education. They predicted, "One day, nurses will be carrying a computer (cell phone) in their pocket to help bedside providers take care of patients."

The folks from WebMD were compelling in their pitch. They wanted our educational materials as content to get started. However, educational material sales were a sizable portion of our revenue. In time, we negotiated a percentage of revenue to AACN in return for them digitizing our materials for the Internet. Suddenly, we were on the virtual world stage with this new company, reaching new audiences.

This meeting proved to be valuable to us in the innovative virtual world. Suddenly, we needed to worry about the value of our virtual intellectual property (an unfamiliar term to me). I worked with our corporate attorney to navigate this different realm. We had a major hospital system buy one copy of ECCO notebooks for a few hundred dollars and digitize them for their several hundred hospitals nationwide. We eventually won a cease-and-desist order to stop them from reproducing our materials. We created pricing structures for hospital systems while also racing to digitize the materials ourselves.

The founders of WebMD were correct in their prediction about cell phones. Today, ECCO *is* available on nurses' cell phones and *remains* the standard for critical care nursing orientation nationwide. This phenomenon spoke to the creativity, drive, and resilience of a national office team working tirelessly to preserve the integrity of the materials while generating revenue to create even more resources. I was proud to lead that effort.

Executive Director

I was the Executive Director of the AACN membership organization from 1997-2000, working my way up through four levels of leadership. While I was in that role, we revised and refined the organization's key initiatives, working in partnership with Sarah, the Board, and the staff leadership team. Once again, I found myself in a hotel meeting room, now with all the leadership team and board members. We were surrounded by flip chart papers covering the walls, scented markers on the tables, and a variety of sticky dots. We worked in groups to evaluate each initiative whether to keep, revise, or sunset. We shed (sunset) the activities that no longer served the organization to funnel time, energy, and financial resources into initiatives to position the organization for the next decade.

I began to study servant leadership, developed by Peter Greenleaf,[43] to manage the organization. It was predicated on the leader serving people to help them elevate their performance and achieve their goals. The cycle is a self-fulfilling prophecy in that the more individuals improve, the more positive they feel about their work. The leader enables this cycle.

AACN celebrated its thirtieth anniversary in 1999. I was honored and amazed to lead the organization that had shaped my practice and life for the past quarter-century. I developed visionary leadership skills and learned how to create an engaging organizational culture.

My responsibilities continued to expand. In 1997, I organized a delegation of 125 critical care nurses for a study tour to Hong Kong and mainland China before Hong Kong reverted to Chinese control. There were shared education sessions between our delegation and the local critical care nurses. Hong Kong had sparkling clean emergency departments with wait times of fifteen minutes. We toured hospitals dedicated to alternative therapies in China.

I served on Robert Wood Johnson advisory boards for critical care medicine. We hosted international congresses for critical care nurses with interpreters and headsets to hear sessions. I made nurses visible through presentations, often to large groups. Asserting myself in front of large audiences required a huge step outside my comfort zone but was fueled by my desire to achieve a goal for the profession or AACN.

Our team advocated for critical care nurses, patients, and families on Capitol Hill in Washington, DC. We wrote testimonies for our national leaders to present to Congress. Sarah, testified in 1995 to the US Congress House Committee on Appropriations, Subcommittee on the Departments of Labor, Health, Human Services, Education, and Related Agencies.

Sarah urged the Committee to fund a pilot research project through the Agency for Health Care Policy and Research (AHCPR) to find the best strategies to implement the Patient Self-Determination Act (PSDA) at the community level. Her testimony inspired approval for an essential piece of legislation languishing on the sidelines of healthcare.

The PSDA passed by Congress in 1991 was a seminal moment for healthcare. Implementation of the law was stalled because there was no plan for the best course of action to reach patients. It required hospitals and nursing homes to advise patients, upon admission, of their right to say their end-of-life wishes through an Advance Directive, which served as a durable power of attorney for healthcare or a living will in case they became incapacitated. The law intended to allow patients to direct their care and avoid some of the excessive life-prolonging treatments often used without regard for quality of life. There was also a great deal of suspicion, particularly from people living on the margins of society, that an advance directive could be used to deny them necessary and lifesaving medical care.

"We can reverse the once irreversible. Critical care nurses know well the suffering, the uncertainty, the guilt, and the incredible difficulty for loved ones when faced with the need to make treatment decisions without the benefit of knowledge of patient preferences." Sarah explained to the Committee.

It was January 26, 1995, twenty-five years since the first Medic One call in Seattle ushered in a new technologically advanced medical era. Rapid cardiac and trauma care improvements using central lines, external pacemakers, dialysis, and left ventricular assist devices enabled us to extend patient lives. The most visible end-of-life-extending challenges, feeding tubes and ventilators, were becoming controversial. As advancements were made, the ever-pressing issue of patient autonomy for end-of-life wishes, which allowed them to control their final days, was more complex than we could have imagined.

The Great Tension appeared again but with a new twist. How can we assure humane and ethical end-of-life care in a healthcare system used to heroic measures that may now be overused, often to the detriment of patients?

Sarah's concern about the PSDA was well-founded. While AACN grappled with end-of-life issues, two high-profile cases including Karen Ann Quinlan and Nancy Cruzan had already made the news. The Karen Ann Quinlan case in 1975 erupted when the 21-year-old took valium and stopped breathing after having several drinks at a party. Paramedics were called, and she was resuscitated, but it was unknown how long she had been without a heartbeat and oxygen. She was unresponsive, considered in a persistent vegetative state, and placed on a ventilator with a feeding tube.[44]

Her parents requested her ventilator be removed because they believed it caused her pain. The hospital was threatened with homicide charges by the Morris County, New Jersey, prosecutor if they removed the ventilator. Hospital officials supported the parent's decision and won the right to remove her from the ventilator. She continued to live, being fed through a feeding tube, and finally died of respiratory failure nine years later at age thirty.

In 1990, Nancy Cruzan clinically died at age twenty-five from a motor vehicle accident.[45] She was resuscitated after fifteen minutes with no oxygen to her brain, which resulted in the loss of brain function. She was kept alive in a persistent vegetative state with a feeding tube for another seven years until the Supreme Court determined enough people who knew her agreed she wouldn't want to live in this condition. It ruled the tube feedings could be stopped per her family's wishes. As these families fought for the right of their loved ones to die without the aid of advanced medical treatment, they faced many court challenges compounding the stress and grief associated with making such a painful decision. These cases also galvanized people between the right-to-life and the right-to-die controversy.

Fortunately, Sarah was successful in her quest to have the AHCPR receive funding for a pilot research project to implement the PSDA, now four years after the law was passed in 1991. She teamed up with University of Southern California (USC) researchers Peter Clark, Susan Evans, and Douglas Shook who created protocols and guidelines to implement advance directives. AACN coordinated the data collection activity. In 2005, AACN published the *Acute and Critical Care Choices Guide to Advance Directives* to assist people in completing an Advance Directive.

Still, it wasn't until 2010 that the Advance Directive movement tried to gain further traction when the Patient Protection and Affordable Care Act (ACA) proposed to close this loophole by reimbursing physicians for offering counseling about end-of-life care through an advance directive. However, this provision was removed from the final ACA legislation after the public feared death panels would decide which at-risk patients would be worthy of medical care.

Today, patients on Medicare are screened for an advance directive at their annual visit with their primary care provider. Patients are routinely asked if they would like to discuss end-of-life care during this visit.

Standing at the bedside of desperately ill patients gave me insight into my end-of-life decision-making. I have a detailed Advance Directive. My family know my wishes: give me a chance if I become unexpectedly ill. If an acute illness or accident requires a ventilator and I have a reasonable chance of complete recovery, I agree to a ventilator for a brief period. My directive has a firm *no* to tube feedings. Ventilators and tube feedings are vital decision points because once they are started, the choice to stop them becomes heart-wrenching. My simple, final directive to my family is, if there is little hope for my definition of quality of life, tell me you love me, give me a kiss on the forehead, and morphine for comfort.

Power of Prayer

Dr. Larry Dossey met with our AACN leadership team. One of our beloved staff directors, Abby, had a fierce recurrence of her breast cancer and she was getting worse by the day. We were beside ourselves trying to figure out how to help her. We sent notes, meals, prayers, and spent countless hours hoping for another remission.

"We are praying for the wrong outcome," he said. "None of us know what is best for her, so praying for her to be healed is not helpful. We want the best outcome for *her*." Dr. Dossey was a respected and treasured member of AACN. His legacy was grounded in his research involving the power of prayer, spirituality, and other non-physical factors to help with complex medical circumstances. He described love or profoundly caring for the person of one's healing intention as a key ingredient in healing.

He offered advice and counsel to a leadership team and national office steeped in grief and mourning. Our precious friend lost her battle with cancer a few days later. It was swift. She fell ill at the NTI in Orlando in late May, and by early July, she was gone. Her loss was deeply felt by staff and volunteers around the country and the world.

Dr. Dossey was the Editor of *Alternative and Complementary Therapies in Medicine*, published by Innovision Communications, a subsidiary of AACN. He was the former chief of staff at Medical City Hospital and former co-chair of the

Panel on Mind/Body Interventions for the National Institutes of Health.[13]

Dr. Dossey offered scientific evidence that prayer worked. Prayer or a prayer-like state of compassion, empathy, and love were the key ingredients to change health outcomes in over 130 controlled laboratory studies. Of note was research from the University of California, San Francisco Medical School. A study of 393 patients hospitalized with heart problems was divided into two cohorts.[13] The first section of patients with only first names listed and a brief description of their illness were enrolled in the intercessory prayer group who received healing prayers from across the U.S. The control group didn't receive prayer. The study was blinded, so neither physicians nor patients knew if they were in the prayer cohort.

The study's inspiring results showed the prayed-for group had fewer deaths, needed fewer medical interventions, and developed fewer complications. Dr. Dossey observed, "If what was being tested wasn't prayer but a modern drug, this would have been heralded as a wonderful medical breakthrough. People would have lined up around the block to get their hands on it."[13]

I was particularly interested in his research because of my involvement as a critical care nurse. All those sleepless nights when my intuition told me my patient was in danger, suddenly made sense. I had dealt with the unsettling feelings by sending healing and comforting thoughts to my patients. I started this practice in my first year as a nurse when I made my night shift rounds. His research confirmed my actions as relevant.

Dr. Dossey's work revealed a finding that caused skepticism in conservative religious groups. There was no correlation between an individual's private religious beliefs and the effect of the prayer. This meant no religion had cornered the market on prayer.[13]

I often said working at AACN was the Disneyland of critical care nursing. Today, it is still one of the profession's crown jewels. It remains so because of the guiding principles and strong values which were part of its foundation. I made a mark on the profession and a real difference in the education of critical care nurses. I am so glad I leaped off that cliff.

In 2000, AACN faced a financial turning point. The Board chose to restructure the national office. I was part of the restructure plan and my position was eliminated. I was offered my prior position as Director of Professional Development, but I opted to leave to find another interesting opportunity.

CHAPTER 13

Amyotrophic Lateral Sclerosis

Director of Patient and Family Services

A family pulled into a precarious parking spot in a busy San Francisco neighborhood where the ALS (Lou Gehrig's Disease) specialty clinic was located. It was 2002. My boss, Linda de Mello, the Executive Director of the Amyotrophic Lateral Sclerosis Association Bay Area Chapter (ALSABAC), observed them with sadness in her eyes.

"We need to write a grant for patient services in the rural areas of our region," she said.

The family parked their modified van and lowered the electronic lift with a power wheelchair to the ground. In the wheelchair was a thirty-seven-year-old man with a tracheostomy, his breathing supported by the ventilator attached to the back of the wheelchair. His brown eyes smiled brightly at me. It was the most movement he had in his body. His loving family had dressed him and carefully positioned him in the wheelchair and driven two-hours from

Monterey to San Francisco for his quarterly clinic visit with the ALS specialty team.

I was the Director of Patient and Family Services for ALSABAC. I attended clinics every Tuesday and Wednesday to support patient and family needs through resources available from the Association.

San Francisco was my favorite city to work in at this point. I lived in Vallejo, across the Bay, so my commute to the city involved a one-hour ferry ride to the Embarcadero. We docked at the famous Ferry Building, which was undergoing renovation to restore it after the 1906 earthquake devastated the city. The clock in the Ferry Building tower stopped at the time the quake hit a century ago. I walked or took the historic cable cars to our office in Union Square. Lunch breaks offered an excellent opportunity to explore the charming city.

I was looking for an organization with meaningful work and a mission of service where I could make a vital contribution after I left AACN. Then, by some karmic magic, I met Linda. I was mesmerized by our conversation in the interview. She was intense, earnest, energetic, and dedicated without question to the organization's mission. Our hour passed swiftly by in what seemed like minutes. We found ourselves building on each other's ideas. She was one of the two most exceptional leaders I had the honor of working with. Sarah was the first.

Linda was known as a dynamo. She had a storied history in education and non-profit circles. She had long advocated for equal opportunities for marginalized people, whether patient, family, or student, in what she called a democratizing process where individuals have equal access to information and connections to university and healthcare systems. Linda holds an honorary doctorate of humane letters from Golden Gate University in San Franciso due to her humanitarian and philanthropic contributions. She was honored by many organizations, including the League of Women Voters, who bestowed upon her the *Women Who Could Be President* Award.

ALSABAC was started by a founder whose wife had succumbed to the disease, but the rapid growth of patient services required the guidance of a seasoned leader. Linda embraced the challenge. She was known to recognize talent and enlist them in a joint venture, an attribute for which I was grateful.

Linda turned to me again. "Phyllis, we must find a way to take these services to our rural areas so these patients don't have to make this long, exhausting trip. And many patients in that area don't have the resources to come to San Francisco."

I nodded. Linda was correct; this was too much to expect of patients and families battling such a tragic disease. I watched as she talked with the patient and his loved ones. I was fortunate to have found her and this organization. Finding the right fit after working for AACN was tricky.

I had written many program proposals at AACN but never a grant proposal. Linda walked me through the process. This was yet another pivot to expand my skill set. She was meticulous with every word, ensuring the intent was powerful and directly addressed the points the foundation sponsoring the grant sought to achieve. We proposed bringing the ALS expert team to the Monterey area every quarter. The hospital there was supportive, and the community had higher-than-average incomes with the appearance of wealth. However, the health disparities, such as access to care, poverty, and lack of medical insurance in the area, were significant for lower-income individuals. The clinic would benefit them most.

ALS is a medically devastating disease and a financially draining one. Medical support at home cost about $200,000/year in 2002. Families struggled to supply life-sustaining equipment to keep their family members alive. The required daily attention was all-encompassing. Spouses left their jobs to care for their loved ones. Children learned to listen to ventilator alarms and knew how to reconnect their family member if the ventilator tubing disconnected from the tracheostomy. Families were exhausted making it through each day, and yet most wouldn't change their decision to keep their loved one at home.

Many patients with ALS are younger than the population in a nursing home, where one might expect ALS patients to be placed. Their minds were still active and alert, so the nursing home solution would devastate them. Our task was to help ease the caregiving burden on the families to the best of our ability.

I empathized with their plight. I recalled the responsibility of caring for my grandfather with brain cancer in 1977. While he wasn't ventilated, we didn't have home technology then, he did require total care supplied by my grandmother, my brother, and me. I knew what it was like to lie beside his bed, listening to his breathing. As with these families, I wouldn't have changed my decision to care for him.

The Monterey Community Foundation funded our grant proposal. We were elated, but now the real work began. We organized skilled professionals already in high demand in San Francisco to take the traveling clinic to Monterey. The clinic featured a neurologist, nurse, speech therapist, physical therapist, social worker, and augmentative equipment specialist with eye-tracking devices that created computerized speech. The clinic worked and took a tremendous burden off the patients and families. We were relieved.

ALSABAC's service area was immense, covering most of northern California. We needed to reach out to other remote areas and stretch the healthcare providers even further.

Working with Linda was a delightfully symbiotic relationship. We supported and pushed each other to higher levels of performance. I handled the patient services and grants, so her time was free to work her magic networking with the San Francisco community. And magic it was. She was so personable, genuine, and compelling; her donation requests were difficult to resist.

My leadership background proved beneficial as I developed programs to help ALS patients and families. I integrated all the insights I had in nursing administration into the organization's mission. I appreciated all too well the issues patients and families face when battling the always-fatal ALS. My background as a critical care nurse was helpful to them. I could walk into their home and help. They didn't have to explain the situation.

Respite programs paid for qualified providers to care for the patient while the family caregiver attended to medical appointments for themselves, grocery shopping, or other tasks to keep the family going. We later added a respite program for children to attend summer camp for a week and just be kids. They could sleep all night and not have to listen for the sound of their parent's ventilator alarm.

The National ALS Association sponsored a lobby day in Washington, DC. Our office brought a ventilated ALS patient in a wheelchair and caregivers to meet with legislators and their staff. We lobbied for extended SSDI benefits for ALS patients without the mandatory two-year wait period. Many ALS patients wouldn't survive the two-year waiting period to collect SSDI. Our requests were met with compassion and interest.

A year later, our efforts succeeded. ALS joined a brief list of diseases as one of the instances when SSDI would take effect immediately after diagnosis, avoiding the two-year waiting period. One other disease included the 1973 decision to include Dr. Scribner's advocacy for ESRD patients to receive immediate benefits after diagnosis.

***

Dr. Richard Olney founded the ALS Center at the University of California, San Francisco, in 1993. Under his leadership, the facility reached the ALS Association Certified Center of Excellence in 2001. He was genuinely committed to a multidisciplinary team approach to ALS care. Patients attending his clinics met with nurses and the specialists who provided comprehensive patient care. He remarked, "Creating the Center was one of my greatest accomplishments."

He served as the Medical Director for the ALSABAC Patient Services Committee. I worked closely with him on initiatives to improve the lives of patients and families. I admired the talented neurologist who was so dedicated to the patients he treated and their families. He was adamant I treat him as a peer, calling him Rick, unless we were in front of patients. I believed referring to him as Dr. Olney was a matter of the profound respect he deserved. A much different dynamic than in 1975 when I would have had to stand when he walked in the room.

A prolific author, he wrote over sixty scientific papers and was world-renowned as an expert in ALS care. His interest in ALS treatment arose when one of his daughter's junior high school teachers died of the disease.

Dr. Olney was a trained psychiatrist, which made him particularly adept at working with patients and families as they navigated the devastating disease. He was fascinated by how patients remained mentally intact even if they lost their ability to communicate verbally or with facial expressions. Dr. Olney shared with patients and support groups, "Everyone dies; people with ALS just happen to know what they will die from."

Unfortunately, Dr. Olney started to observe stiffness in his right leg in 2003, and soon, his muscle movements and coordination were becoming compromised. He was first diagnosed with a protruding disc in his spinal cord. He underwent surgery but soon began to perceive his symptoms were getting worse. He believed he might have ALS, but more testing revealed more back problems, and he had two more surgeries. By mid-May in 2004, his right arm was now affected with mild stiffness and slowed reactions. He gave himself a standard test for ALS—counting how many times he could tap his fingers in 10 seconds. From experience, he knew he could usually tap sixty-five times, but now he had slowed to fifty-five.[46] He knew he had ALS at that point.

Dr. Olney disclosed his illness to the ALS Center team and then had the challenging task of informing the patients and families in the clinic. Since there is no known cause or cure for ALS, he was concerned patients and families would fear it was contagious, which it wasn't. Dr. Olney resigned from his leadership position with the Center but continued to give many interviews with national news media to promote awareness of the disease.

Dr. Olney died in 2012 at sixty-four. He was one of the few patients who lived so long with the disease. He will be remembered for his dedication to patients and families dealing with ALS. His commitment to excellence in patient care, clinical research, and his advocacy contributed to people with ALS living longer, with better quality lives. Dr. Olney's legacy included important discoveries, promising targets for future research, and more clinical trials than ever in California.[46]

CHAPTER 14

American Cancer Society

Executive Director

I was looking for work in Michigan, where my family relocated. I needed to find a new job that was as meaningful as working with ALS patients and families. I began my role as the executive director of the American Cancer Society East Michigan Service Center (ACSEMSC) in Flint, Michigan in December of 2008. It was at the height of the Great Recession, with auto plants closing, the major employers in the area.

One of my first duties was to review the office lease, due for renewal in 2009, that the attorneys at the corporate office sent to me. I couldn't believe what I was reading. *If a cure for cancer is found or it becomes a chronic disease, and the services of the ACSEMSC are no longer needed during this lease, the owner shall release the ACSEMSC from the lease obligations.*

This was the first time I saw such language in print, much less in a lease. Attorneys were not known as inspirational, so this clause stopped me in my tracks. *Were we close enough to a cure or treatment that would make cancer a chronic disease?* Our fight had been so focused on a cure for decades, a chronic illness was a more realistic goal.

As I noted before, President Richard Nixon declared war on cancer to conquer the disease. He signed the National Cancer Act into law in 1971, around the same fertile time in medicine that Medic One started. Thirty-seven years later, I was reading our lease saying that cancer may become chronic in the next five years.

Cancer was an unwelcome visitor throughout my life. From the first patient I visited as a candy striper, to my grandfather's death from brain cancer, to working with families of children with leukemia at Fred Hutch, to the death of our beloved director at AACN from breast cancer. Now, as the Executive Director, I hoped to contribute to improving the lives of patients and families affected by cancer.

This was an arduous task. The Great Recession of 2007-2008 ravaged the country for over a year. Flint, Michigan, was one of the most devastated areas. In my first few months at ACS, I received several angry calls from community members who were furious I took a good paying job from a man who could have supported his family. I had no words. I felt like I'd traveled back thirty years, when women weren't welcome in executive positions.

Unemployment in Flint was one of the worst in the nation, as most of the auto plants closed in the area. When people lost their jobs, they also lost their health insurance. The Affordable Care Act was several years away as a safety net for health insurance.

Fundraising events were our primary source of income. Our service center managed three Making Strides Against Breast Cancer walks and fourteen Relay for Life events each year. It was a rigorous fundraising schedule in an area where snow covered the ground from October to April.

Our staff was small, with only five event coordinators and two patient service specialists. On the other hand, our cadre of volunteers was quite large and propelled these events into successful fundraisers. During my tenure at ACS, we reached our $1 million per year fundraising goal despite the recession. We turned our office budget from a deficit to positive.

This career pivot taught me how to motivate a large cohort of volunteers. The volunteers were tireless. They, too, were on a mission to end this dreaded disease. They found tracks at local schools for Relay for Life events and set up individual campsites around the theme, *Fight Back Against Cancer*. Families created teams with a team member always on the track during the twenty-four-hour event. There were motivational speeches and ceremonies. Relay for Life events were exceptionally moving and physically exhausting for everyone involved. I attended each event to support the staff and volunteers while walking laps with patients and families. Survivors were celebrated with a victory lap and, after dark, a Luminaria ceremony and lap honored those we lost to cancer. I bought a luminaria for my Grandpa Harold and walked the lap in his honor at every event.

I marveled at the dedication of the volunteers. They worked year-round to raise money, secure sponsorships, and investigate a myriad of intricate details to make the events exceptional. Many had the time to dedicate to these efforts because they were laid off from work when their auto plants closed. Some were cancer survivors, while others were currently battling the disease. Several were losing their battle with cancer.

A few deliberately decided to forgo treatments. I spoke with Jeff, a laid-off auto worker as we walked a couple of laps together. "How are you doing, Jeff?" I asked softly. "Your wife shared that you were recently diagnosed with pancreatic cancer. I was sorry to hear the news."

"I'm not going for treatment," he replied.

"That's a serious decision. May I ask what brought you to that point?"

"I don't have health insurance," he explained. "I would need to sell my house in a severely depressed housing market to afford care. I'd rather make sure my family has a place to live after I'm gone."

I was stunned and saddened by this reality. "I am so sorry to hear you had to make that difficult decision."

"At least I can raise money to find a cure for someone in the future," he said as we finished our last lap together. I hugged him before he returned to his family.

In 1971, the five-year survival rate for cancer, with only eight drugs to treat the disease, was 50%. Over fifty years later, it approaches 69% for all cancers with an arsenal of over 640 drugs. The most recent data compared 1975 to 2022 for specific cancers. The brain cancer my grandfather died from made marginal improvements in five-year survival rates during this period, from 0% to 8%. The children with leukemia dramatically improved, from 33% to 87%. The breast cancer my colleague at AACN succumbed to showed progress from 75% to 90%.[47] These are remarkable statistics. I was again embedded as a leader in a region's communities, working with health disparities, and making a difference in patient and family lives.

I loved this meaningful work, but my family was relocating once again. At ACS, I started mentoring others in leadership positions so I would have a qualified person to replace me and be able to move on in peace. The larger question for me was, what new challenge do I want to embrace?

Part VI

Nursing Research - PhD

CHAPTER 15

Doctoral Program

In 2005, I returned to school for my doctorate in human development at Fielding Graduate University. It was the perfect fit for me. Decidedly self-directed, with faculty accomplished in their field and interested in mentoring a new generation of leaders dedicated to social change. My study concentration was in Transformative Learning for Social Justice. Transformative learning is accomplished by challenging our assumptions and perspectives of life events. These are complex but critical skills for working with vulnerable populations.

Working as a nurse for over thirty years, I witnessed the effects of healthcare disparities based on socioeconomic factors. Longer waits in the ER, missed diagnoses, dismissed symptoms, and a lack of essential human connection by some healthcare professionals toward patients from marginalized groups contributed to my angst about the system. I wanted to be part of the solution.

My committee chair was a Fulbright Scholar whose academic interest was intersectionality, the study of how complex, overlapping categories of gender, race, and class merge to create systems of oppression and discrimination. She was brilliant, impatient, and frustrated at my lack of academic capability. *Wasn't that why I was pursuing a doctorate?* I wrote in the language of healthcare and business. She didn't trust mainstream big business, especially healthcare.

I tried my best, but she tossed my dissertation draft back at one of our meetings. "Your proposal needs more work before I'll read it." Her eyes held a hard gleam when they met mine. "This is a part-time gig for me, I don't have time to hold your hand."

I was crushed and had a sick feeling in the pit of my stomach. I'd spent months creating that draft. She went into a tirade about how I didn't understand intersectionality and until I did, there was no point in her reading my work. But she was my committee chair. *I* was paying full-time tuition. She needed to help me.

"Will you help me understand the basic premise of intersectionality?" I pressed.

She gave me a five-minute lecture on what it was and why I should care. The lecture ended with, "You need to study this more," as she got up to leave.

***

If one believes in the Saturn Return promising life upheaval when the planet returns to the same position in the sky as when I was born, then my Saturn Return appeared with a vengeance. The years preceding my twenty-eighth birthday were tumultuous and collided with my rewarding professional life. I lost my beloved grandfather from a brain tumor. I experienced my fourth miscarriage, which led to the breakdown of my ten-year marriage. Finally, a close female colleague supported me through this turmoil. This relationship grew into a romantic one, marking my transition to a lesbian. I had nothing to lose by taking big leaps, but the details about these events are for another book. I am eternally grateful my career was my safe harbor during this time.

***

I was a closeted lesbian as the assistant administrator at SVH. I worried that hiding an important aspect of my personal life impacted my authenticity with my team. I had practiced disclosing my sexual identity at the UWMC. When I arrived at AACN, I was still selective. I was candid with the people in the office but guarded my disclosure with the members of the Board, who were from areas all around the country, some from very conservative states. I convinced myself I had a right to privacy. But my conscience was pestering me that it was secrecy. The internal conflict set off a decade long internal struggle. *Was this secrecy or was it privacy?*

I started researching lesbian executive disclosure as a hobby when I worked at AACN. This should say a lot about me when research is a hobby. I submitted a paper to a think tank conference and presented my work, *Dimensions of Organizational Cultural Diversity for Lesbian Executives* at a seminar at the Sixth Annual International Critical and Feminist Perspectives in Nursing Conference, sponsored by Carlow College in Prouts Neck, Maine.[48] It was my first national presentation about being a lesbian. I wish I were confident, but my voice was hesitant. Sometimes, it shook, and I rushed my presentation with a monotone voice. I was so nervous, yet it was well received. The discussion was spirited, and the participants offered diverse opinions and more ideas for me to consider. I was relieved and energized.

I persevered deeper into my dissertation, diving headfirst into the literature about the topic. I had a great deal of intersectionality experiences in my life as a woman and a lesbian. I sat with my findings and applied them to my life, then rewrote my dissertation proposal.

"This is a little closer," she said grudgingly.

My cohort of doctoral students met to share our dissertation topics for feedback. When I shared mine about lesbian executives disclosing their sexual identity, the response stunned me.

"Being lesbian is too widely accepted for this to be relevant," one student said.

Another argued, "This is old news."

Yet another piped in, "I agree, this study is unnecessary."

I reminded myself of my fellow students' backgrounds. They were well-educated, liberal, and lived in progressive larger cities (Fielding is a national university with international cohorts).

"I respectfully disagree," I argued. "It's still legal to be fired for being gay in thirty-three states. Besides, we can't even legally marry." It was 2004, a decade away from the legalization of same-sex marriage.

I felt vindicated when I conducted my interviews. The lesbian executive participants, some from Fortune 500 companies, offered detailed accounts where they were marginalized or had to use care disclosing details about their personal lives.

One participant, Susan, described her experience. "With every generation, another layer peels back, but I honestly could tell you that if I worked in the Midwest, we wouldn't be having this conversation. I wouldn't even be admitting that I was out. I would be living a closeted life. I'm lucky to live in the gay haven of San Francisco."

When describing her lesbian identity, she said, "You have to get to a point where you're comfortable with it in your soul."

Another participant, Emily, was disappointed her sexual identity was still a concern. "At this point in my career, I was like, 'Oh gosh, I only have a year left to work, and this is still an issue.' I still must stop and think about it. But that's part of what you carry being gay in this society. It's disappointing. We're not to a point where it's okay to be out."

She noted that being an executive made a difference. "It was probably more of an issue when I was working my way up through the organization, being concerned about how it impacted my promotions if people knew or if I were openly gay." Emily explained. "But now that I'm here, it doesn't matter much."

After my data collection, I took a brief break to attend an intensive experience endorsed by Fielding. The Highlander Research and Education Center is a cultural center and social justice training school in rural New Market, Tennessee. It was the perfect respite while I pondered my data.

CHAPTER 16

Highlander Intensive

Fielding's mission drew me to the university. Their emphasis on transformative learning and social change inspired me and offered tools to make change in my small corner of the world. The four-day Highlander Intensive I attended in 2007 with half-a-dozen other students changed my social justice work. Myles Horton and others founded Highlander in the 1930s to address inequities in the workforce. By the 1960s, the Civil Rights movement, particularly the commitment to end segregation, became the focus of their mission under the premise that peaceful protest creates a space to work through conflict together.

Highlander's peaceful protest teachings were controversial. Over the years, the Center endured decertification by the state, a devastating arson fire, and a lack of local support because of their civil rights efforts. Unable to find local labor to rebuild after the fire, the Center staff purchased a vacation home kit. The rustic octagon-shaped structure was perched on a hill in the Great Smokey Mountains. Within the walls of that simple octagonal great room sat a circle of a dozen oversized wooden rocking chairs reminiscent of southern porch rockers.

When I entered the octagon, I felt an overwhelming sense of heaviness in my chest, which sparked my desire to understand what happened in the room. Our facilitator explained that Highlander had provided education and strategies for peaceful protest during the Civil Rights movement. Martin Luther King and Rosa Parks sat in the very rockers where we sat. I read Rosa Park's autobiography and was inspired by her small stature yet quiet persistence in her quest for equality. I sensed a kinship with her and a responsibility to contribute to social justice work.

Intensive was the perfect word to describe our experience. We slept on bunk beds and were called to simple, southern, communal meals by a dinner bell outside the dining room. We came to challenge our assumptions and discover strategies to support our social justice work. My focus was on the lesbian experience because of the overlay of gender and sexual identity.

Spirited discussions marked most of our time together as we found common ground and worked through our differences in the Highlander spirit. I was surprised to hear from a few fellow attendees they believed the plight of lesbians wasn't as dire as it once was, that being gay was more accepted, and that women had made strides in gaining rights. I found myself defending my stance, as I had earlier at Fielding. These discussions opened my eyes to the importance of suspending judgment, listening, and seeking to understand a person's pain around injustice rather than dismissing them.

As if that wasn't life-altering enough, we had one more surprise ahead of us. Our last night was emotional. We'd shared so much of our deep longing for social justice and faced our biases together. At dinner, the facilitator told us that special guests would join us for our evening session. We wondered who it could be.

When we entered the octagonal room and headed to our rockers, we saw an older couple, the man leaning over his guitar. Guy and Candie Carawan welcomed us and played folk songs about peace. As the evening progressed, our facilitator explained that Guy sang *We Shall Overcome*, the anthem of the Civil Rights movement, during many critical historic moments alongside Martin Luther King, Jr. He didn't write the song but lent his talents to a cause near to his heart. He closed our evening together, asking us to sing the song with him and Candie. I did my best but did so through tears in my eyes so thick I could hardly see. The reverence of the week crashing around me, the history of Highlander, our shared and sometimes contentious conversations, and the sheer magnitude of the moment was overwhelming.

***

I returned to Fielding with a renewed sense of purpose, determined to overcome the resistance from my dissertation chair and some of my student colleagues. A three-person faculty committee critiqued our dissertations. One of the committee members specialized in the research process, and she willingly took me on as a project. Under her watchful eye, my proposal took shape. After a LOT of arduous work, I was ready to defend my completed dissertation in a talk open to the entire university, a couple dozen people attended. Immersing myself in one topic for years gave me enthusiasm and confidence in my work.

The title of my dissertation was *Identities at the Intersections: Lesbian Executives Experiences with the Management of the Disclosure of Their Sexual Identity in the Workplace.*[49] (Academia has such catchy titles.) It is housed in the National Library of Congress with our country's other doctoral dissertations.

It was a qualitative study based on the experiences of lesbian executives from around the country, defined as having a leadership position on a board of directors. The study sample had a diversity of race, ethnicity, religion, and ableness. The participants navigated an invisible identity in a visible organizational position, and their lesbian identity remained a subtext that permeated their relationships with others.

The most significant finding was that most participants believed being a woman was the visible, primary identity they most attended to in the workplace. However, several observed their lesbian identity also played a role. "Visual cues lessen the burden of coming out repeatedly with new people. It's torture to come out again and again," a few participants noted. The need for authenticity was a force in managing their sexual identity disclosure decisions.

The findings opened the door for more discussion about intersectionality encounters with each of the identities I studied. My work also described some microaggressions designed by society to keep a person from reaching their full potential. It was my introduction to microaggressions, or "death by a thousand cuts," which I experienced in my younger days when lesbian relationships weren't considered "real" relationships.[50]

My dissertation defense went very well. After a grueling four years, in November 2009, I was officially *Dr. Phyllis Heintz*. I published an article based on my research findings in the journal *Career Development Quarterly*.[51] It was my published national coming out story.

After successfully defending my dissertation, one of my fellow students suggested I submit my doctoral findings as a session for a conference. My presentation, *The Balancing Act: Preserving Personal Authenticity in the Workplace*,[52] was accepted for Out and Equal's national conference. The non-profit's mission was to help executives advance best practices in diversity and inclusion and promote workplace equality for LGBTQIA+ (lesbian, gay, bisexual, transgender, intersex, queer/questioning, asexual) employees.

For the second time, I took the national stage to present my work about being a lesbian executive. I approached the stage with a different mindset than I had fifteen years before at the Critical and Feminist Perspectives in Nursing Conference in Prouts Neck, Maine. I was self-assured, and I spoke confidently about my journey as a lesbian executive. In the early days of my career, I decided to be intentionally vague about my sexual identity as a leader, which caused others to question my authenticity. Leadership positions are extremely visible, and I am transparent. If I evade a topic, it is evident on my face, triggering people to doubt my truthfulness and credibility. A deal breaker for a leader.

Presenting to an audience of like-minded LGBTQIA+ leaders was energizing, and the audience members engaged in an energetic discussion about how we could balance our identity, remain authentic, and thrive in our positions. My *secrecy vs privacy* debate was solved; the answer was about me becoming authentic with my identity.

Part VII

California State University
Bakersfield

CHAPTER 17

Faculty

I started looking for a job when my family relocated to Bakersfield in July 2010 with my shiny new doctorate. Excited to discover my next opportunity, I applied to every hospital in town. I had just one interview with one of the larger hospitals in the area. The Vice President of Human Resources entered the room and announced, "I'm only interviewing you as a favor for the Chief Nursing Officer, her friend recommended you. You're way too qualified for the Quality Improvement Director position and you would never be considered for bedside nursing."

I had pursued a PhD for my own personal interest. I hadn't considered how it might affect my future employment opportunities. I'd always found exciting work as a nurse. I was discouraged; apparently, this small town had no positions for doctorally prepared nurses. I was too young to retire. I had student loans in repayment, adding another layer of anxiety.

One morning, I came out of the shower and looked in the mirror. A red, blistered line in the shape of a lightning bolt traced the nerves on the left side of my face. It stung after the hot shower. I was so stressed that I developed shingles. Luckily, I was treated quickly, including a trip to the eye doctor to discover I had a lesion in my eye. I was put on Acyclovir, and the lesion resolved without incident. Still, I learned a valuable lesson about keeping my emotions and stress in check. I tend to obsess over things, trying to figure out how to fix an issue.

Bakersfield was the home to one of the smaller campuses in the California State University (CSU) system. The nursing department had a Simulation Coordinator position open. I applied and received an invitation to interview with the Search Committee. As I stepped into the front office of the nursing department, the administrative assistant asked, "If you aren't selected for this position, would you consider something else?"

Oh no. I hadn't even met the committee yet and was asked about a different position. Of course, I responded, "Yes." The interview went well, and I fit well with the faculty. Days turned into weeks, then a month.

I picked up the phone to call the Department Chair and reached her voicemail. I left her a detailed message, hoping to hear something back soon. About an hour later, I received a call from Human Resources. I wasn't selected for the position. I was shattered. It was an entry-level position requiring a bachelor's degree in nursing. Evidently, the University wasn't interested in doctorally prepared nurses either.

Half an hour later, I received another call. It was Debbie, the Chair of the nursing department. She described the intricate job search process involved at the university. I was familiar with the complexities of university management from my time at UWMC. Debbie explained that my skills and expertise were beyond the position I applied for, and she hoped I would be interested in a faculty position.

My heart raced as she described how the department approached teaching. I was invited to join the adjunct faculty at CSU Bakersfield (CSUB) for the winter quarter. I was elated. I enjoyed teaching, and CSUB was designated as a Hispanic Serving Institution (HSI) with 62% of the student body of Hispanic heritage, the perfect match with my doctorate.

In my first meeting with Debbie, I liked her. She was dynamic, complex, engaging, and passionate about teaching and nursing. She described the faculty, how the department functioned, and the students in the program. I could co-teach a Lifespan Development course to pre-nursing students. I immediately accepted, and she introduced me to my mentor Karen, the psychiatric nursing instructor. Debbie left us to talk.

Karen and I made plans for January, with each of us assigned to develop specific elements. We met a few more times before winter term started, and Karen asked me to teach the first day of class. I taught critical care and leadership to staff nurses at UWMC two decades earlier. We used a lot of paper and Kodak slides. Nurses either called us on the phone or showed up in our offices. Now, we had PowerPoint slides and the BlackBoard online learning system.

All students had laptop computers, and we communicated via email or in person.

I was so nervous that first class, ensuring I covered every point on each slide. I'm sure it was as tedious for the students as it was for me. Karen's gentle guidance helped me relax, and I began to weave a story, rather than lecture, for the students. I included some anecdotes so the material wasn't so dry. She was a terrific mentor and, coincidentally, an LGBTQIA+ ally, supporting queer students in crisis. I talked about my personal life with her, and she is a dear friend even today.

I was offered a full-time faculty position as a lecturer for the next academic year. I eagerly accepted. I felt at home at the university and enjoyed the students and faculty.

The first year of full-time teaching was intense. I had five classes each quarter. During those first two years, I spent many hours preparing my lectures, creating the BlackBoard virtual spaces, and learning the workings of academic life. In addition, I completed a two-hundred-hour nursing refresher course, including eighty hours of unpaid precepted nursing practice in a hospital unit. The California Board of Registered Nursing required a refresher course if a nurse was away from the bedside more than five years.

A year later, the Robert and Edith Cochran Endowed Chair for Gerontological Nursing, a tenure-track position became available. I again marveled at the synchronicity of my professional life. One of the reasons I wanted to become a nurse was to care for my aging grandparents. I applied.

The interview process for tenure-track positions was rigorous. I met with the department search committee, the dean, the grants office, and the provost. I ended the day by presenting a one-hour lecture open to the entire campus. My presentation was evaluated by all attendees with the feedback provided to the search committee. I prepared a talk about geriatrics titled *The Silver Tsunami*,[53] illustrating the most current and future trends in the care of the older population. The presentation went well because of my passion for the subject and the inordinate amount of time I spent preparing for the talk. I was awarded the position.

One of my priorities was to establish my research agenda. I selected ageism, using my interest in intersectionality. The CSUB Institutional Review Board (IRB) approved my proposal, allowing me to interact with human subjects.

I engaged the entire sophomore nursing class to collect data. Each student took the IRB training and interviewed a woman over fifty using a fixed set of questions related to women's ageism experiences with health professionals. I also taught the junior research class, so those students completed data analysis. The study sample was representative of our diverse student body. We found participants alleged instances of ageism, sexism, racism, and homophobia throughout the study sample, primarily from medical assistants who had the least education but spent the most time with patients.

Several students in my research class were published in journals with me, then presented podium and poster presentations at regional and national conferences. It was a real benefit for those students to have research activities on their resumes when they applied for nursing jobs after graduation.

My faculty role allowed me to give back to the profession. It didn't pay well, but it was immensely rewarding. The students got the benefit from my experiences through the stories I shared. We could think through some of those same challenges together. I hoped this would help them with problem-solving in their careers.

The spring quarter of 2014, I was the nursing instructor charged with teaching the first-year nursing students how to become nurses. We were at our noon conference. With a mischievous smile, Stacie pleaded, "Dr. Heintz, tell us another story, pleeeease!" She was young and playful, always finding a way to stall returning to the unit. The other students nodded. She was the brave one who spoke for the group.

"Alright, one more, then it's back to the unit." I said.

"Ken told us about the LVAD (left ventricular assist device) supporting his patient's heart function," I began. "The LVAD Ken saw today is the size of a large iPhone. When I worked at the University of Washington Medical Center in the late Eighties,

LVADs were just invented. The LVAD I worked with was the size of a refrigerator.

"It took three nurses to walk the patient. One nurse rolled the large unit on wheels. One nurse managed a pole on wheels with all the IVs keeping his blood pressure stable. And one nurse helped the patient as they walked. I'm always amazed at how much healthcare has advanced in my lifetime. It's fun to imagine how it might change during your career."

The students were near the end of their first year, attentively studying their textbooks, examining the faculty's every move, and timidly showing up at patients' bedsides. Looking around the conference table, I could tell they were mentally and physically exhausted.

They worked hard in nursing school, putting in long hours of study the night before they arrived at the unit for their twelve-hour shifts. They met with me before their 7:00 am shift started to review their pre-work for the day. Each student prepared papers on pathophysiology, nursing diagnosis, details about every medication the patient took, and formulated a care plan for the day. These documents were their ticket for admission to work twelve hours tirelessly, for free, under my watchful eye, the anxious questions from patients and family, and the sometimes-skeptical looks from the nursing staff. The students were naively auditioning for future jobs at the hospital after graduation.

If their homework was incomplete, they were sent home and unable to participate in the clinical practice for the day. They got a zero for their grade and may have only one episode per quarter, or they failed the course. If they failed the course, they must petition the department chair to be readmitted and wait another year until the course is offered again. If they failed two courses at any time, they were dismissed from the program and must find another profession.

Transferring to another school wasn't an option because they had to give a letter from the department chair declaring they were in good academic standing, which they were not. That was a lot of pressure for young nineteen or twenty-year-olds, but it's required for them to assume the role of a nurse who often held a patient's life in their hands. One error from lack of knowledge or preparation could result in a patient's death. None of these students were in that category.

Working with this group of ten students all year was my joy. They had unique life experiences and diverse backgrounds in age, race, ethnicity, gender, and religion. Yet they converged as a cohesive team capable of managing groups of students and patients.

As faculty, we were supposed to be neutral about our observations of students, using grading rubrics and clinical ability to measure their progress and assign grades objectively. As a person, I couldn't help but reflect on our year together and smile to myself. I wasn't supposed to have favorites, but this was my favorite clinical group.

Ted was an older, tall, husky man, a military veteran with the stamina and rigor required of a hero who served our country. As a medic on the front lines, he had more real-world experience than some civilian nurses. He towered above my 5-foot-2-inch frame yet was so kind and respectful of my role as his leader, responding, "Yes ma'am, no ma'am" when I quizzed him or gave instructions.

Ken was self-assured and slightly older than the other students. His winning smile charmed the nurses. Despite my attempts to allocate new clinical skills evenly among all the students, the nurses found interesting procedures for him to perform. He called me "the Ninja Professor" because I silently stepped as if on cat's feet, an innate habit from my years in nursing.

Alma was a bright, quiet, shy young woman. I gently but firmly coaxed her to speak up. She shared, "In my family, young women were to be inconspicuous." We discussed how we were sometimes conditioned as women not to be the first to speak. I explained, "We are the first line of defense for patients. Physicians may not be aware of a profound change in a patient's condition. Rounding on patients goes so fast. If we are not quick to speak out about a patient issue, it may be overlooked, with dire consequences."

Alma worked hard to heed my advice. She engaged with patients and families more often, answering their questions and offering reassurance. She communicated with the nurses more directly. One day, she asked her patient's nurse, "May I call my patient's physician about a change in my patient?" The nurse working with her sat beside her, listening as she made the call.

Another student, Erika, offered in a quiet, almost reverent voice, "Dr. Heintz, I wish I could be like you when I grow up." She was a beautiful young woman who was even more beautiful in her heart. Erika lived in a multigenerational household. She was the first in her family to attend college as her relatives carefully saved to send one child to college at a time. She was also one of the smartest in the class of fifty-five students. This was no small feat since the grade point average of students accepted to the program was above 3.75.

I am not sure I could get into nursing school today. I was a solid B student in high school, with a 3.0 grade point average. As a first-generation college student, I charted my own course alone. I improved with each college degree, but that initial step up in post-high school education was crucial to my professional growth. My work as a faculty member was important because my early college experience inspired me to work with underrepresented or forgotten students.

I looked at Erika. "You already *are* just like me."

She continued. "We learn so much from your stories, and sometimes we can see ourselves doing just what you did." *Hooray! That was my goal.*

Students from the foster system may be suddenly sent away from their foster homes when they "age out" on their eighteenth birthday, leaving some abruptly homeless. The foster family no longer received payment for their care, and the trauma of realizing money was the only reason the family took them in was a double assault on their hearts. I helped them and other students find scholarships and offered moral support to help them navigate work while going to school, which is challenging in the nursing program because of the clinical shifts they had to complete.

As the out lesbian faculty member in the department, LGBTQIA+ students knew they could talk to me about their concerns. CSUB had a *Safe Ally* program where faculty learned about resources and strategies to help these students navigate the challenges in their lives. I took the training and placed the Safe Ally triangle on my office door.

College is ground zero for young people coming into their sexual identity. I listened as they struggled with their sexuality, especially those who were sexually assaulted. The early twenties are a treacherous time for students, especially women and marginalized people.

A clinical unit lends itself to intimate life conversations. Over the years, a few students found me in private moments on the unit and asked, "How did you know you were gay?"

I replied, "It was an evolution. One day, I fell in love with a woman. It felt like I won a game of Tetris, and the world started making sense." More was said, but most students silently took that in. I offered, "You're welcome to call me anytime to talk, even after graduation."

Several of these students had already faced their share of trauma or adversity, from abuse at home, poverty, or discrimination. In an average class of fifty nursing students, statistically, ten would have been sexually abused as a child, five would love someone of the same sex, five would be food insecure and need the food pantry on campus, three would be housing insecure sleeping in their cars or couch surfing, and a whopping thirty of them—more than half—would be marginalized based on their race or ethnicity. Some would be marginalized for their gender. In nursing, men may have a problem when patients refuse to have a male nurse, especially in obstetrics. I faced two of these adversities myself.

I wanted my students to develop perseverance and confidence to prevail. I used Appreciative Coaching with them. We worked together to focus on their strengths and apply those behaviors to develop new skills. I encouraged my students to "run their own race," learn how to face their fears, believe in themselves, and listen to their intuition to develop a strong inner voice. When they were hesitant, hands shaking before they started their first intravenous line, I gave them a mantra actors use in the theater: *Commit to the moment*, to provide them with the courage to swiftly perform the procedure. I believe we learn more from our failures than our successes and, in the process, grow as humans and nurses. Most times, when I was knocked down, I found a way to get back up through grit, perseverance, and sheer determination. I ultimately found myself in a better place.

When I took students to our Alzheimer's Day Care in Bakersfield, I taught them therapeutic communication with clients along the dementia spectrum. While it didn't happen often, sometimes a client would become agitated, pacing, and yelling. Their skin was hot to the touch from their high metabolic rate. Our usual tactics to divert their attention were no longer working. It was frightening to students when clients in crisis paced and yelled; calming them became a nurse's challenge. One of the first tricks I learned at the daycare was to sing *You Are My Sunshine*. I would start singing softly, "*You are my sunshine, my only sunshine. You make me happy when skies are gray...*" while walking with the client. In time, the client would join in the song and become calmer. It was almost magic. I taught my students that song. Yes, I had to teach them the song since some of my students were born around the 9/11 attack on the World Trade Centers. Most never heard of it. At first, it was awkward; they were not used to singing, but they caught on when they saw how well it worked.

My work ethic was a model for students. No amount of telling would have the same impact. I always logged at least 11,000 steps by noon on clinical days. I taught, monitored, coached, and encouraged each student. I modeled talking with patients, families, doctors, and colleagues while supervising students completing tasks. I stressed the importance of integrity, defining it as what we do when no one is looking. We are alone with patients and their medications, including narcotics. Our own moral compass guides our actions.

But now, the students were weary and slumped in their chairs, finishing their lunches, and presenting their patients to the group. They still had another five hours left before they summarized their day on paper and gave a report to the oncoming shift of nurses and me. They needed another bit of rest and could use yet another story to encourage them to the finish line. I shared one of the stories in this book ... they must have heard all of them over the last year. They appreciated hearing the real-life stories about being a nurse, the exhilarating, and heart-wrenching moments. They asked questions and offered insights I hadn't considered. In short...

They inspired me to become a better nursing professor.

***

I immersed myself in my second year of teaching as the Endowed Chair for Gerontological Nursing. I hit my stride as a faculty member, taking my turn at chairing different committees. I resurrected grant writing efforts that laid dormant for over a decade. I became the department champion for online teaching as it was introduced to the campus.

During a faculty social event at the end of the school year, one of the faculty members said, "You should be chair someday."

I enjoyed leadership positions. Instead of planning care for a patient, I designed the working environment for the organization I led. In my mind, the skills were transferrable.

It meant a great deal to me to be faculty. Universities are steeped in tradition. Each fall, a hopeful group of new students would swarm campus. We welcomed them with a Convocation ceremony where each student received a pin from the University. Parents pinned their students, but CSUB had some students without parents. Some were released from foster care, others emancipated early, and some whose parents didn't have time off from their jobs. As faculty, we filtered through the crowd to find students to pin. Tears welled up in my eyes as some students would shyly ask me to pin them. I welcomed each one with a hug.

Commencement held the same emotional meaning for me. I always kept sight of the significance of sitting in my faculty regalia on the dais. As the nursing students approached the stage, my faculty colleagues and I left our seats and walked to the line of graduates waiting to receive their diplomas. Tears, hugs, and high-fives abounded.

CHAPTER 18

Intuition

If you loved bedside nursing, why did you step away to leadership positions?

People sometimes asked why I pursued other areas of practice. The answer was profoundly personal and seldom talked about by nurses. For this reason, I have no idea how many nurses this experience affects. The phenomenon to which I refer is intuition. It was a sense of knowing different from individual or experiential knowing. Spencer[54] explained, "Intuition is your soul whispering the truth to your heart and hoping that you hear."

Nurse theorist Patricia Benner[55] said it is "Based on the knowledge we gained as expert nurses where we processed multiple pieces of data to guide our practice." I believe it arises from empathy with my patients. I persevered as I learned to trust my intuition enough to listen. My strong intuition and empathy served me well as a nurse.

The most troubling for me was the feeling of death surrounding someone when I met them. It wasn't a vision but a visceral sensation in my core, a heaviness in my heart, an unsettling sense something was wrong or, as Obi-Wan Kenobi observed in *Star Wars*, "A disturbance in the Force." I couldn't see the outcome, but it was a disquieting sensation that someone would die. The sensation wouldn't come often, but sadly, it was right more than wrong. The sensation may come from meeting the patient or even a family member.

When I worked in the Pheresis unit at Fred Hutch, I rarely met the children who were our patients. I worked with their siblings and parents. Sometimes, the sensation arose in my first encounter with a family member, and the feeling was unshakable for a long time. I had this reaction from my first meeting with Brittany's family. This was the most disturbing element about the sensations; enough of them came true.

I also had this intuition as a critical care nurse. In that setting, I sometimes sensed the patient's health would decline. As a young nurse, I didn't fully understand the sensation. Sometimes, I believed I was doing something wrong and worried about what that might be. In most of those instances, the patient's vital signs were stable, and there was no sign anything drastic was imminent. After a few cases of the patient going into cardiac arrest soon after I sensed those feelings, I decided next time I would call the physician. I prefaced my comments by saying, "The patient's vital signs are stable, but I have an uncomfortable feeling they might deteriorate." Most physicians were courteous and listened, recommending I let them know the second anything happened. A few came to check the patient as soon as possible. Even fewer got angry that I had disturbed them. A few I remember vividly.

In one instance, when working at SVH. I was caring for a patient in critical care for a few days when, one afternoon, I had a terrible feeling of dread when I looked in his room. I checked him thoroughly and called the physician. "Dr. Roberts, all Mr. Evan's vitals are stable, but something doesn't seem right to me."

"I'll be right there," he said.

I returned to the patient's room. The patient arrested as Dr. Roberts walked in the door. After we resuscitated Mr. Evans, Dr. Roberts said, "I'm grateful you called." He didn't know how grateful I was that he believed me. The patient survived.

The sensation that something was wrong with a patient was so overwhelming that, as a bedside nurse, sometimes I couldn't sleep. I agonized, and as this feeling wouldn't leave, I began to send reassuring feelings toward the patient and family to comfort them and myself. If the connection with them was so strong that it affected me this way, then maybe my kind energy shining back could reach them. I like to believe this was so.

I had one patient, Jack, call the hospital soon after his discharge. He experienced a heart attack and was critically ill for a week. I was his day nurse for most of his hospital stay when he was so sick. I talked to him, as I did all my patients, while he was ventilated and unresponsive. I talked about the weather, the news, my cat, what I fixed for dinner, and some way to keep his mind stimulated despite being in a coma. He slowly began to recover during my week off. When I returned, I transferred him to step-down care.

It was Jack on the other end of the phone in the ICU a few months later. "Phyllis, may I come take you for coffee? I want to hear more about my hospital experience."

I had no idea he remembered who I was. He was extremely sick most of the time I cared for him. I was intrigued, so I agreed. He met me at the hospital during one of my rare lunch breaks. I told the other nurses Jack wanted to talk to me. They were also interested and offered to cover my patients for me.

When I stepped into the cafeteria, I looked around. It was Jack who recognized me. He looked nothing like the patient dangerously close to death for whom I had so vigilantly cared. He was slim, clean-shaven, in jeans and a flannel shirt. His thin blond hair was neatly combed, and his bright blue eyes were smiling at me.

"Thanks for meeting me. I recognized your voice from when I was so sick. I didn't know who it belonged to, but you returned and cared for me as I got better. I knew it was you."

He asked, "Could you please talk about my time in ICU? How sick was I? When were you most worried about me? How did you know I would be all right?"

I told him the honest details, among them, "You were extremely sick, and we cared for you with intense concern. Your numbers were near death for several days."

"Thank you for filling in the blanks for me. By the way, how is your cat doing?" His eyes twinkled at me as he laughed.

"Oh, you remember what I told you when you were on the ventilator?" I was surprised.

"Enough," he laughed.

As I talked with him, I realized I never had that ominous sensation of death when caring for him, even though he was riding the razor-thin margin of it.

In all my decades of practice, only one other person, a sophomore student nurse, Jeanette, ever talked to me about her encounter with this phenomenon. She was worried and spoke in hushed tones, fearing the other students would hear her. We met in a quiet area of the hospital. Jeanette was petite in stature but firm in her presence. She was visibly upset and looked down as she was talking to me. "Dr. Heintz, sometimes when I care for people, I can tell they will die. I have Mrs. Lopez, and I know she's going to die." She was sobbing at this point.

Mrs. Lopez was extraordinarily ill but not outwardly in imminent danger of death. "It's very upsetting, isn't it?" I asked.

She lifted her head with tears running down her cheeks and stared at me with a puzzled look. I asked her questions about what she witnessed or how she felt, trying to help her describe what she experienced. For me, it was a feeling. I didn't have visions. It was the same for her.

"How will I be a nurse if I can't handle this?" she asked.

"A little at a time is how. Do you still want to be a nurse? If you don't, now is the time to find another career path," I offered.

"No, no, I still want to be a nurse." She was adamant.

I sat on the windowsill next to her. "Here's the thing, I know exactly what you're feeling." She looked at me through her tears.

"Jeanette, I've never shared this with anyone. You're the first person I've met who shares this phenomenon ... or at least is brave enough to discuss it."

"What phenomenon?" she asked.

"The ability to sense when someone is going to die. I can't tell when or how, but with some people, I can sense they will die."

She looked at me, incredulous. I shared with her the sleepless nights, the uncomfortable but incalculable feeling. I revealed *the dance* I would do with my career in the early years when I was engaged in caring for some of the sickest patients. Whenever the nightmares and uncomfortable sensations started, I changed jobs. I sought safety in outpatient dialysis, teaching, or research.

I returned to the bedside for one more round in the ICU at SVH. That was my last full-time direct bedside care position after eighteen years of *the dance.*

Nurses from all disciplines experience trauma from a variety of sources. Our nervous systems are constantly on alert, responding to codes and emergencies. We navigate environmental factors, exposure to diseases, chemicals used in medications, and violence from patients or visitors. Our emotional well-being is tested by sudden deaths, especially with children, and the most devastating of all, rare medical errors we cause. Navigating this trauma is the stuff nightmares are made of, or we wall it off as an act of self-preservation.

Jeanette intently listened.

"Do you feel a patient's experience in your body?" I asked.

She looked down and quietly said, "Yes."

"And you still want to be a nurse?"

"More than anything," she said in earnest.

"Well, let's strategize." I offered.

We talked about how to approach *the dance* for the next several minutes. "Try to find someone you trust in whom you can confide when these situations arise. Think about the line in the sand that will cause you to shift your career focus." I suggested.

I encouraged her think about future career options. "You might want to seek an advanced degree for more mobility."

I closed by asking her to stay connected with me throughout her career. We hugged and went back to the unit. We never spoke of the episode the remaining two years she was in the program, but we knowingly smiled at each other, having shared that secret. I received an email from her about five years later:

Good afternoon, Dr. Heintz!

I'm sending you this email to let you know that I often think of you and want to remind you how thankful I am for everything I learned from you during my school years. Thank you for helping me be the nurse that I am today. Thank you for teaching me, sharing everything you know, and listening to me when I needed it the most. When I think of that one inspirational teacher that I have had and that I will forever be thankful for ... that is you :)

I remembered many patients and students I was graced to care for and teach. After writing the first draft of this chapter, I retrieved Jeanette's email, which she sent several years before. I replied to it. I told her what I was doing and asked how her career was going. I received a joyful email in return.

What a lovely surprise! I must admit my eyes got teary as I read your email. Tears of joy for recalling all the beautiful memories of you that I hold dear in my heart. When I think of that special and inspirational teacher...your beautiful smile and spirit come to my mind.

I'm still practicing as a Registered Nurse but recently decided to go the holistic route. Over the years, my patients have taught me so much. I loved bedside care; however, I didn't feel the freedom to attend to the deepest needs of my patients. I saw and felt that their suffering was much more profound than their physical symptoms. It was precisely this deep connection with them that was so difficult yet so meaningful in many ways.

I went back to school, took a few courses in Holistic Nursing, and got certified through the American Holistic Nurses Corporation. This and other complementary medicine therapies have allowed me to express my renewed thoughts in healing and feel so grateful for my journey. I continue to learn every day.

Jeanette nailed it. She embraced her gift and ran toward it. I was so proud of her and wondered what would have happened if I had the strength to embrace the gift and run toward it rather than do *the dance* I chose. I will never know, but instead, take solace in the memories of my remarkable career full of contributions I am grateful to have made to nursing.

CHAPTER 19

Department Chair

Over the next several years, I built my tenure credentials. I served as assistant Chair for a few years to learn the leadership and accreditation aspects of the department. The Chair position was three years, renewable once, and then term limits required that we find another Chair. After Debbie reached her term limit, in 2016 I became department Chair.

I was so excited. I immersed myself in academic life and enjoyed good working relationships with the staff, faculty, students, the rest of the University, and the community. All my prior practice and education was a plus for the position.

Of course, there were challenges, and I played the hand I was dealt. I learned to do so at SVH. The University changed from a quarter to a semester system in the first year I was Chair. A fourth of the faculty resigned or retired in protest, not wanting to redesign their courses for semesters. A treasured faculty member lost her husband to cancer at the same time and chose to resign. She needed a fresh start in life; we understood and wished her well. She was an influential informal leader, and her absence left a void in the department. The administrative staff moved on to other positions. The Dean, Assistant Dean, and Provost also turned over.

The leadership chain from the administrative staff, to me, to the University leadership were new to our positions. I created a mantra to sustain us through this challenging transition. When times seemed hopeless, I advised our team, "the only way out is through," meaning we might get lost in the weeds of uncertainty and grief, which were the dark side of achieving our goals. Still, when we walked through the process together, step by step, we accomplished our objectives. It was genuine team building, and the next academic year began with solid faculty and staff.

The California Board of Registered Nursing (BRN) conducted the five-year continuing approval visit during the spring semester, which placed a lot of pressure on me as Chair. I created a large document describing our educational efforts, procedures, processes, and outcomes. The report was accompanied by a classroom filled with banker's boxes showing evidence supporting my claims, such as examples of graded student work and data about first-time pass rates for the registered nursing state board exam. The visit went well, and we were approved for another five years with a glowing report. My knowledge of drafting massive reports and detailed inspections at SVH served me well.

I enjoyed the position and was awarded early tenure. I continued writing grants to support our underrepresented student population in our medically underserved area. Most of the students remained in the community after graduation, increasing the pool of nurses. Granting organizations were impressed how many graduates remained in Bakersfield. This was the perfect use of my doctorate to create social change in our community.

A person's zip code can determine two key health outcomes: length of life and quality of life. Length of life measures items such as deaths before age 75. Quality of life looks at a broader range of data, such as health behaviors (smoking, diet, alcohol, and drug use), clinical care (access to and quality of care), social and environmental factors (education level, employment, income, family and social support, and community safety), and the physical environment (air and water quality, housing, transit).

Kern County, where Bakersfield is located, had vastly different health outcomes than San Luis Obispo County, only two hours to the west on the Pacific coast. Kern County ranked 53/58 counties in California for length of life. San Luis Obispo County was 13/58. Quality of life differences were even more staggering, 57/58 for Kern County, while San Luis Obispo County was 7/58 counties.[56] Kern County was ground zero for poor health outcomes in California.

This wasn't just an academic exercise. We all should understand the zip code dynamic and care about the plight of our fellow humans in those disadvantaged areas. Clean water and air are a necessity and significantly affect health outcomes.

Our grant efforts focused on increasing access to high-quality medical care by educating nurses. The grant presentations in Sacramento in front of the Office of Statewide Health Planning and Development (OSHPD) Commission were highly competitive. The proceedings were recorded and formal. The first presentation I made to this daunting commission was nerve-wracking. My voice shook, but we were awarded funding for two years. I taught grant writing skills to many faculty so we could write more grants. We were gaining traction as a team, and the future looked bright.

By the time I retired, I had raised $1.85 million in grant funding to support the education of underrepresented nursing students. Fielding's mandate to become *a scholar-practitioner* echoed in my mind. I was grateful I applied my social justice education to make a difference in my small corner of the world, one patient at a time, one student at a time, one day at a time.

I moved back to Seattle when I retired to reunite with my family after twenty-five years in California.

Part VIII

Life Beyond the Bedside

CHAPTER 20

Medical Reserve Corps

Registered Nurse Volunteer

It was the first day of spring in Seattle in March 2021, and rain came down as I walked past the totem pole at the Northwest hospital entrance. The COVID-19 pandemic raged on for over a year, decimating the economy and people's lives. My demographic group was now eligible for vaccinations. The city was on shelter-in-place orders for over a year, so my ability to travel and visit friends was severely curtailed.

Today, I stood in the same hallway for the vaccination clinic where I'd once stood as a candy striper on the medical surgical unit fifty-two years ago. Now considered the "old" hospital, it was used for various community services. It was surreal leaning against the hallway railing as I did so long ago. I reflected on my incredible journey, how blessed my career was, and how it let me follow my heart. I was grateful I made a difference in the lives of so many patients and families.

As a candy striper, I was excited about becoming a nurse yet filled with trepidation because I had no idea how to become one.

Eventually, I figured it out and found the professional settings where I was joyous, creative, and surrounded by loving and energetic colleagues. When I found those settings, I fulfilled my potential and felt aligned with my purpose. I used my intuition to contribute to the healing of others.

I arrived at the vaccination clinic early, wearing my mask while I waited in a short line of people to be screened, and checked in for their vaccine. A can with the label *clean pens* on the reception counter caught my eye as the young woman behind the glass divider explained, "You'll be getting the Pfizer vaccine, not Moderna."

"It doesn't matter, as long as I can be vaccinated," I replied.

COVID-19 was still a new disease. While it was believed to be spread by respiratory droplets, there was some early evidence that the virus might live for a brief time on inanimate objects. Severe cleansing protocols were put in place throughout the country. No one touched anything in public spaces, using elbows and other means to press elevator buttons.

When it was my turn, a nurse led me through rows of small cubicles with chairs for patients and tables for vaccinators. She said, "We administer around six hundred vaccines daily in this clinic." I marveled at the precision and attention to infection control as so many people were ushered through the process.

Afterward, as I sat in chair #10 waiting for the required fifteen minutes after the vaccine to make sure I didn't have a reaction, I reflected on what this day meant in the context of the over fifty years I stood by patient bedsides.

Now, I could safely take a vaccine that, by all measures, was a medical miracle. Most vaccines take ten to fifteen years to produce. The COVID vaccine was developed and moved through the mandated clinical trial procedures required by the Food and Drug Administration (FDA) in record time, less than a year. It was cleared for emergency use authorization in December 2020 in much the same manner as Zofran was cleared for widespread use when I was at Fred Hutch. With a worldwide collaboration based on the fifteen years of research into coronaviruses of other types, some associated with the common cold, researchers were able to ascertain this virus's structure, genome, and replication. Cancer and HIV research also contributed an extensive knowledge base about genomic sequencing, making the structure of the virus more easily identified. This vaccine wouldn't have been available so quickly if the pandemic occurred three years earlier. We would have faced years of development.

The nation faced the daunting task of vaccinating most of the adult population. Vacant parking lots in colleges and transit centers were converted into mass vaccination clinics since people were sheltered at home. There was almost no traffic as the pandemic raged on. Interstate 5 was eerily empty for the first time since it opened in 1964. It seemed like an apocalypse.

I was so fascinated by the speed of vaccine development and rapid deployment that I did what I knew best. In the spirit of remembering my career roots as a volunteer, I joined the county Medical Reserve Corps for medical professionals to help with the drive-through mass vaccination clinics to contribute to the pandemic mitigation efforts.

When I stepped into the vaccination tent, it felt like home. Four other volunteer nurses were there, and we instantly formed a team. We spoke the same nursing language and had the foundational education in the universal procedures of injections and patient care. We understood we could trust each other's skills. We were given a quick information session by the clinic manager, who advised, "We can get ten doses out of a vial. Mix the vial thoroughly before drawing up the dose, but don't shake it. Today, we're giving Moderna vaccines, so draw up 0.5 ml in each syringe. Only draw up what you think we'll need for two hours. We must keep the vaccines at the proper temperature to remain effective. Don't leave them out of the special freezer for over two hours."

We quickly divided tasks. I went to the observation area. I marveled at how my career was symmetrically bookended by volunteering at the bedside (and car side) while significant medical advances were evolving. A tad longer than a year from the country's first death from COVID-19 in Washington State, I was walking a line of cars using my nursing expertise to observe newly vaccinated people for fifteen minutes.

I instructed them, "Stay in your car, keep the car in park, and the door unlocked in case we need to reach you quickly. Honk your horn if you don't feel well."

With so many to be vaccinated, I was soon reminded of the starfish story. A man watched a boy throwing starfish back into the ocean. The man said, "There are hundreds of starfish. You can't make a difference!"

The child replied, "I made a difference for that one," as he tossed another starfish in the water (adapted from The Starfish Thrower)[57]. I greeted each client in the vaccine clinics with a smile, thanked them for coming, and thought about the starfish story.

We vaccinated over five hundred people each day. Most were grateful for the chance at everyday life again. Some were emotional, as I was when I received my vaccine. A few with a history of vaccine reactions were parked near the command tent for a closer 30-minute observation.

One young woman fainted in her car. We promptly laid her car seat flat, put her feet on the dashboard, and prepared to call Medic One if she didn't improve. Luckily, she quickly regained consciousness.

Fifty-two years ago, an emergency medical services system was not available to activate, much less a highly skilled medic unit available within minutes with sophisticated equipment and highly trained paramedics to help her. I stood by her, absorbed by the magnitude of living in Seattle. Suddenly, the expertise of those Medic One responders brought a tear to my eye.

CHAPTER 21

Reflections on a Career

No one understands a patient's experience better than their nurse. No one can understand a nurse's encounters better than another nurse. This phenomenon is purposeful, foundational, and universal. Each of us comes to the profession with our own life story, yet we unite when we don our scrubs and step foot on the unit. Nurses are called to alleviate pain and suffering, care for us when we are most vulnerable, and guide us through life's most precious moments – our first and last breaths.

My nursing career trajectory followed distinctly different paths with multiple pivot points when I took advantage of the opportunities for clinical specialization, leadership, and professional growth. I worked my way up in organizations through hard work and persistence to obtain executive positions.

I want to say my career path was calculated, planned, and strategic, but it wasn't. Instead, I followed my passion for different practice settings. Our profession navigates an array of complex factors such as the aging of our workforce and the resulting shortages, burnout, with economic changes putting financial pressure on healthcare settings. We experience concerns about workplace safety in terms of exposure to violence and infectious diseases. Flexibility is the hallmark of a fascinating nursing career.

As the Palm Reader observed those decades ago, it was like falling off a cliff. I recognize now that I trusted myself and the universe that I would be caught, so I didn't try to crawl back up the cliff. The growth was in the fall.

I appreciated the role synchronicity played in my life. My career evolved in tandem with the most significant advances in medical history as I worked alongside true pioneers. It supplied unmatched opportunities to be present for bedside moments, which were nothing short of miraculous. For me, nursing was a science practiced as an art.

Why would anyone want to be a nurse? My Grandma Phyllis asked me that question when I said I wanted to be a nurse. For most, there are practical reasons. Nursing is an honorable profession with elevated levels of honesty and ethics. For two decades, Gallup ranked nursing as the most trusted profession. Nurses are in high demand with flexible shifts and good wages to support middle-income families. For some, income stability is enough, but to be candid, there isn't enough money to be a nurse for the money alone.

For others, nursing is a calling to humane service at the bedside of people during the most vulnerable time of their lives, those who need us for protection and advocacy. No matter why one becomes a nurse, we are guardians for patients and families as both navigate the razor-thin line between life and death, health and sickness, or joy and grief. For me, nursing was a calling, my passion. I responded to the calling at fifteen, and fifty years later, I responded to another call to begin an enjoyable retired life. It was pure grace.

I can't tell you how many lives I've saved. Nurses don't count those things for cocktail party conversations, it would be unprofessional. I also can't tell you how many family members' hands I have held, nor how many patient's eyes looked into mine, the last eyes they ever saw. I was in the room when we saved those who, by all measures, had no chance, while others who should have survived didn't despite our best efforts. I passionately believe there is a power greater than us that sometimes guides the outcome.

My fifty-year nursing career was captured in moments, often life-altering moments. I acquired endearing memories and insights. At the same time, I learned valuable lessons from bedside conversations with physicians, nurses, patients, families, and students. Nurses were instrumental in the work of brilliant physicians and their remarkable innovations. We had the luxury of applying early medical advances as part of everyday medical care.

Standing at bedsides with the physicians in this book was transformative. Their intensity, passion, intelligence, and kindness permeated each patient's room. They taught, coached, celebrated successes, and deeply felt the losses. Their standards were high, almost unreachable, but I worked hard to meet those expectations. My most significant contribution to their efforts was caring for patients so effectively that I could help anticipate their clinical course. I diligently cared for patients, collecting a dizzying myriad of patient data, before computers, to prepare for possible outcomes. That exhilarating and rewarding attentiveness made me a cherished part of these historic teams. It was fate, my life path brought me to this time in history. When medical miracles were taking off, my career path followed. It was very Forrest Gump-like.

I realized the magnitude of working with these remarkable pioneers several years into my career. In many instances, I called physicians in the middle of the night because of grave circumstances. Why wouldn't I call Dr. Hickman to troubleshoot the patient's Hickman line? Who else but Dr. Scribner would be declotting a Scribner shunt? I cherished the opportunity to work one-on-one with them during those midnight hours. Watching them as they bent over a patient, quietly solving the problem while reassuring the patient and family, are still vivid and cherished images in my mind. With these pages, I captured intimate perspectives as mere snapshots of nursing practice over half a century. I examined these medical advances through the lenses of the scientific, social, ethical, and economic impact they contributed to modern healthcare. I described my career pivots to explore new challenges, avoid burnout, and find ways to keep my passion for the profession alive.

I embarked on this project after years of teaching nursing students at the bedside and telling them stories of my career. Those students were like me: the first generation in their family to navigate college, respond to a calling, and enter a profession they *believed* they understood. The students were fascinated by my anecdotes. I realized there was a treasure trove of lessons to be shared and a compelling history to capture for an essential era in medical modernization. I was a hero to them, yet I did not perceive myself as a hero. While it was flattering to hear students say they wanted to be like me, I did not want to leave them with the illusion that my path was easy for fear that any hardship in their lives would discourage them from achieving their goals.

Nursing was the stable foundation to achieve my vision of service. My career drove me to persist through tough times. As a nurse, I could chart my course and expand my abilities to become the most vital force in my career. I re-energized myself over the years by pivoting to switch specialties, learn innovative technology, and mentor others. I realized the most fulfilling paths I took were unexpected. My career was shaped by personal development and self-discovery for a calling that deeply resonated with me. I learned life lessons I may not have otherwise encountered. The grace I received from my profession filled my life with meaning, joy, and happiness.

Challenges and disappointments humbled me and fueled my doubts and fears about my abilities. Mentors through their support and my perseverance, allowed me to emerge transformed.

I captured a front-row seat to these medical wonders, collaborating with innovative physicians through the hope and heartache associated with professions that genuinely cared about patients and families.

In many ways, I am still a fifteen-year-old candy striper at heart, in awe of the physicians and leaders who perceived some promise in my work ethic, compassion, and nursing expertise. I am eternally grateful for their trust in me.

My childhood dream of becoming a nurse became an anchor for my life. It allowed me to thrive as an adult. My wish is that people affected by adversity find the perseverance to manage their own health or forge a meaningful path forward in nursing for themselves.

CHAPTER 22

Legacies

I was an RN for forty-eight years, with a front-row seat to patient care in some capacity for fifty-three years. Now, we are amid another burst of astonishing advancements in medicine. I retired in 2023. We'll see how long it lasts.

I was awarded Associate Professor Emerita in Nursing from CSUB when I retired. Emeritus status is an honorary title to recognize distinguished teaching and outstanding service to students and the University. I was one of only ten people to receive the honor in the forty-five-year history of the nursing department. I continued to teach part-time due to the shortage of nursing faculty. I was called upon to cover faculty emergency leaves and help with special accreditation projects. I soon realized that Emeritus status was like fairy god mother status, an enduring spirit of service. Not too shabby a legacy for a teenager who almost failed high school chemistry. I was beyond honored the department nominated me for the award. Yet, finding meaning and purpose in my life after retirement loomed before me. I wondered, was this just the beginning of something greater than I can imagine now?

As I wrote the finishing touches on this book, CSUB celebrated fifty years of graduating nurses. I joyfully attended. Two former students, now faculty, caught me for a photo under the colorful blue and yellow balloon arch decorated in a nursing theme.

After the photo, one of them turned toward me with watery eyes. "I have fond memories of you as a teacher and I am trying to be like you."

My eyes blurred as I tried to hold back tears. How often do we get to hear about our legacy while we're alive? I can rest easy. The next shift of nurses is now at the helm of the profession.

Innovator Legacies

I would be remiss if I didn't share the traits of the brilliant innovators in this book. Their legacies are shining examples of perseverance and clinical expertise. The qualitative researcher in me scoured the literature to study them. I was curious about the attributes these innovating physicians had in common. I combed various articles and awards about them. I collected the descriptors ranging from a Nobel Prize award to lifetime achievement recognitions. The work of Dr. Scribner, Dr. Cobb, Dr. Thomas, and other innovators opened the door to saving the lives of individuals with acute and chronic life-ending diseases. Sadly, not every life could be saved, and the pressing ethical question of whether a poor quality of life should be maintained began to surface in the late 1970s and continues to today.

Physicians as a group are knowledgeable and skilled, yet there was something particularly compelling about these physician innovators. To assign a ranking of importance of one over another evades my imagination since each of their enduring contributions changed the lives of millions of patients worldwide for decades to come. All the innovators, both physicians and thought leaders featured in this book shared some unique characteristics, primarily in clinical excellence, personal traits, and vision.

Clinical Excellence

Clinical excellence was the cornerstone of the physician innovators' work. Most were known for their lofty expectations and dedication to bedside practice. Though they spent thousands of hours refining their skills, their proficiency flowed through them. Since their clinical expertise was second nature, they focused on their patients. Indeed, most innovators were known for a fierce devotion to their patients and expecting excellence from the nurses standing beside them at the bedside. Their lifelong curiosity about their specialties was infectious. They exuded a groundbreaking spirit that inspired those around them to join in their journey.

Nevertheless, these innovators avoided being blindsided by enthusiasm and the need for consensus. They remained skeptically inquisitive, true to their foundational training as rigorous scientists. Once satisfied that they had found a safe, reliable, and practical innovation, they zealously shared their knowledge.

Personal Traits

What personal traits sustained the physician and thought leader innovators throughout their thousands of hours and decades of practice? Their innate qualities of being bright and energetic were qualities that undoubtedly sustained them through the rigors of medical education or the demands of leading complex organizations. What made them unique was their passion for solving a problem of significance to help a specific patient population, such as patients with end-stage renal disease, leukemia, heart disease, or ALS. Their unrelenting obsession with finding solutions to thorny problems gave them the courage to take risks when others told them their innovations would fail. Notably, each physician had at least one skeptical colleague who publicly proclaimed that their innovation would fail. The dedicated perseverance of these physicians resulted in millions of lives saved from various medical conditions over the past six decades.

The thought leader innovators led complex organizations dedicated to such daunting tasks as supporting the education and advocacy of nurses who care for the critically ill or improving the lives of terminally ill ALS patients. The thought leaders in this book were my heroes who created trust with their followers, were transparent, and inspirational about their vision.

All the innovators held personal values to sustain them in their careers. They had integrity, an inviolate necessity when conducting clinical trials on human subjects. Moreover, their humility was a trait that fostered collegiality with other professionals on their teams, encouraging open dialogue and idea sharing. Lastly, compassion for their patients was one of their most endearing personal traits. They deeply felt every clinical success and every patient lost.

Vision

Finally, all the innovators showed a profound ability to create a vision for solving some of the most wicked problems plaguing patients affected by severe and life-ending conditions. Published accounts noted that the inventions the innovators envisioned were grounded in a calling to serve humanity by improving the quality of life for patients. After extensive experimentation and reflection, they would take a leap of faith based on the best clinical evidence their innovation would work.

The innovators displayed remarkable resilience to skeptics, partly because they could rely on their exacting clinical expertise or leadership acumen. As their careers progressed, when it was clear they were at the pinnacle of their field, most repaid the accolades they received by serving as role models and mentors for others. The U.W. SOM is now a research powerhouse built on the contributions of these incredible individuals.

Part IX

Taken for Granted

CHAPTER 23

Precious Medical Marvels in Peril

Nurses play a vital role in sustaining the momentum of innovation; however, the burnout of healthcare professionals in general and specifically for nurses, threatens the future of healthcare in the U.S.. We delivered these miracles, yet we may choose other career paths because of the growing headwinds to our practice. These are systemic problems linked to *The Great Tension* without simple solutions, and they compromise our precious medical resources.

Despite the profound breakthroughs in technology and treatment, the healthcare landscape has shifted in ways that make sustaining these miracles uncertain. Sadly, these once-celebrated medical miracles are under increased scrutiny and threatened by extinction.

Over the past decade, there has been a steady regression as medical advancements we take for granted were called into question. Reduction of emergency medical services, vaccine hesitancy, and preventable harmful behaviors jeopardize our system. This regression is exacerbated by challenges such as economic strain from rising costs on the healthcare system and societal skepticism toward medical progress.

Our complacency, lack of support for medical science, and misinformation fuel mistrust, slowly eroding the accomplishments of the last half-century. Our hard-fought battles for medical advancements are in jeopardy. Life-saving expertise becomes undervalued, overused, or threatened due to misuse of medications, lack of trust for scientific rigor, and citizens' lack of understanding about how complicated and fragile our medical achievements are. There is a false sense of security that we can roll back the assaults on our bodies for poor lifestyle choices, while those with a genetic predisposition for these diseases must play the genetic hand they were dealt. We have enough headwinds to a healthy life due to genetics; we don't need to further fuel our body's decline with unhealthy lifestyle choices.

Emergency Medical Services - Medic One

Even our precious Medic One system is in jeopardy of being defunded by the smaller counties surrounding Seattle and I imagine around the country. Outlying county officials believe King County could also cover their service area. Distance, time to reach patients, and finite resources limit that plan's viability. The public either fails to remember or is too young to know the heartbreak of losing loved ones because there was no rapid response to common emergencies, such as heart attacks, before the pivotal year of 1969. At the time, the only choices were to call a mortician or the coroner.

Now the Fentanyl and opioid crisis compounds the problem by diverting valuable EMS resources to respond to drug overdoses to administer Narcan and provide life support. As a critical care nurse for decades, I can count on less than one hand the number of times I administered Narcan. This should not be normal practice. Narcan is now stocked in drug stores and grocery stores. Responding to overdose calls puts patients in peril as EMS services are not available for other medical emergencies. The Fentanyl and opioid crisis and the resulting dependence on extreme Narcan usage points to a public health crisis.

Finally, one of the grass roots, invaluable parts of the EMS system, volunteers, is in danger. Rural areas do not have a sufficient population or tax base to support a paid EMS. Volunteer firefighters and first responders in rural areas are aging out of the volunteer force. These volunteers are a crucial lifeline and recruitment efforts are essential. I fondly remember the volunteer fire fighters at SVH. They knew their neighbors' medical histories and responded within minutes to distress calls, delivering the patients quickly to our hospital.

Vaccine Hesitancy

Unfortunately, the COVID-19 pandemic and subsequent vaccine initiatives became politicized then cast doubt on common vaccines used for decades. The angst escalated as the lay public grew frustrated by nuances in policy shifts in the CDC's approach to the virus which increased the momentum of the pushback against medical miracles. People were divided between believing the science about the disease, its spread, and the public health efforts to fight the virus against the notion that the disease messaging was a hoax or blown out of proportion. This last belief resulted in a reluctance to take the vaccine by a sizable portion of the population.

By mid-September 2021, just a year-and-a half after the shutdown of the nation and six months into the vaccination program, deaths from COVID-19 surpassed the death toll from the 1918 Spanish Flu epidemic, which was previously the most significant viral loss of life in the U.S.. When the Spanish Flu devastated the nation, we didn't have ventilators, critical care units or specialists, infectious disease experts, testing ability, and decades of cancer and infectious disease research to draw upon to create an effective vaccine in less than a year. Medical care had advanced dramatically since 1918. Yet, due to the political division around the disease and vaccines, many people refused vaccinations and needlessly died, leaving families devastated and some children orphaned. If the polio epidemic of my childhood had been politicized in the same way, we would still be battling the disease today. We must learn from history.

Soon, another wave of a virus mutation took hold and started causing deaths among younger people under forty and children. Rationing of critical care and hospital beds started in some harder-hit states because the hospitals were full of unvaccinated COVID-19 patients with the new Delta variant. Some of my colleagues reported a few patients breathlessly whispering, "It's still a hoax," as they were intubated.

The surge was another public health crisis. Hospital beds were full, and morgues were overflowing. Bodies were stored in refrigerated trucks. Once again, as with the HIV pandemic, nurses stood at patients' bedsides, holding their hands, and caring for them as they took their last breaths.

Families were not allowed in the hospital to curb the spread of the disease. Nurses held iPads for patients as families tearfully said goodbye to their loved ones. These heart-wrenching scenes played out daily and began to take their toll on even seasoned nurses.

Two states, Idaho and Alaska, started "crisis standards of care" (rationing) for their entire states. This put all residents, regardless of vaccination status, at risk for being a Do Not Resuscitate patient without their consent. Medical resources such as critical care beds, ventilators, and dialysis were rationed for the first time since the 1960s when rationing was needed because the technology for dialysis was new and we didn't have enough equipment. This crisis was quite different from the prior dialysis rationing. Now, care was limited because unvaccinated patients overran the healthcare system.

New variants kept emerging, yet I continued to show up in those parking lot clinics to vaccinate one person at a time. It was the only thing I could do to tame my frustration about the low vaccination rates and contribute to a solution.

Nurses and physicians were exhausted. People with non-COVID emergencies were dying because hospitals were overcapacity and there were insufficient beds to accept them. The news reported a vaccinated man with a heart attack unable to receive care. The hospital he presented to was overflowing, and the staff contacted forty-three other hospitals with no room to accept him. He died waiting for a bed.

Having come of age as a nurse when science radically improved people's lives, it was disturbing to witness this dynamic unfold. Trying to find a way to change people's hearts and minds was even more frustrating. I can personally attest to the effectiveness of the CDC in protecting the public's health. I have over four decades of nursing experience and weathered two epidemics without a health issue, solely because of the research and protocols the CDC had in place to protect me. Science is data-based. Human interpretation fluctuates. Responsible use of science requires critical thinking and investigation.

Tragically, life expectancy in the US declined by 1.5 years from 2019 to 2020, the most significant drop since World War II, when the decline was 2.9 years.[62] The decrease was from the COVID-19 pandemic death toll. The weekly deaths from the most vulnerable adults, those ages 65-80+ showed dramatic changes from 119 deaths per week in that age group in October 2021, down to 8 deaths per week in April 2023. The vaccination program improved the health outcomes even for those who declined the vaccines.[59] We must continue our efforts to vaccinate most of the population. This includes the usual vaccines for measles, mumps, and rubella, among the other common vaccines. We are starting to see an increase in diseases we had nearly eradicated.

Eventually, the pandemic took more than a million American lives. Yet, it heralded another wave of medical innovation we hadn't seen in fifty years. The discovery of mRNA from innovations in advanced cancer treatment and immunotherapy were now used in vaccines. Without the coronavirus vaccines, millions more lives would have been lost.

Vaccines in Cancer Treatment

"It's stunning," said Barney Graham, a key researcher in developing mRNA vaccines, "The pace of advancement is in an exponential phase right now."[63] The coronavirus vaccines were at the forefront of this new wave. Many cancers, often believed to be life-ending, may now be treated with mRNA discoveries. The funding for these advancements coincided with the Human Genome Project in 2003. Just like in the late 1960s and early 1970s, government investment in NIH funding fueled the rapid progress of medicine, this time creating mRNA tools.

Vaccine research may be the next breakthrough in cancer treatment. Cancer vaccines are designed to shrink tumors and stop the diseases from returning. Cancer cells often hide in the body, but the new vaccines activate a person's immune system to find and fight the cancer cells using mRNA technology like the COVID-19 vaccines. Dr. Nora Disis of U.W. Medicine Cancer Vaccine Institute described the technology: "If you saw an activated T-cell, it almost has feet. You can see it crawling through the blood vessel to get out to the tissues."[64]

By 2021, some cancers were now considered chronic conditions, a true miracle. It was fifty years since the National Cancer Act was passed in 1971. The death rate from cancer declined considerably. I took a beloved family member to his oncologist appointments at Fred Hutch. He battled kidney cancer for twelve years and his current course of chemotherapy was no longer working. We were prepared for unwelcome news. The oncologist explained, "Your cancer has become a chronic disease, and you will likely pass away from some other condition."

I couldn't believe what I was hearing; a little more than a decade after signing the ACS East Michigan Service Center lease with the chronic disease/cure clause, my family member was living proof of our progress in conquering the disease. The oncologist said, "We will try some new targeted therapy drugs to keep your cancer in check. It supercharges your immune system to respond to the cancer and has fewer side effects to improve your quality of life."

Preventable Harmful Lifestyle Behaviors

Up to now, *The Great Tension* between healthcare finance and quality patient care was beyond our control as nurses and patients.

Massive healthcare systems controlled the delicate balance between patient needs and finances to meet those needs. However, now our systems strain under the sheer number of patients presenting with diseases resulting from preventable harmful lifestyle behaviors.

The cascading effect of sedentary lifestyles and our diets laced with ultra processed foods escalated in my lifetime. The good news is that both risk factors are in our hands if we take responsibility for correcting our habits. We are at a tipping point with our medical care. Research funding is declining while our life choices implicated in chronic diseases are left unchecked. This is both expensive and tragic for our society and sadly leaves few financial resources to assist those who live in poverty to obtain preventative measures such as healthy food and clean water. The cycle of poverty is a complex social determinant of someone's ability to lead a healthy life and a predictor for poorer health outcomes and premature death.

The consequences of unhealthy lifestyle choices deliver patients in life-altering crises to our emergency department doors, pleading, "can't you fix this?" in response to a devastating diagnosis. The eroding of U.S. healthy lifestyle choices results in obesity, which places individuals at risk for heart disease, diabetes, and a host of other problems related to the strain on the human body.[58] The correction will take generational change for years to come, much like the efforts to curb tobacco use starting in the late Sixties. We eventually dropped the rate of smoking in half over two generations.

The most stunning aspect of the nursing bedside refresher course I took in 2011 to become clinical faculty at CSUB, was not the change in the patients' physiology, their breath and heart sounds hadn't changed. It was the shift in the magnitude of the diagnoses we were treating compared to when I last worked at the bedside. In 1975, when I started practice as an RN, the rate of type 2 diabetes in the US population was 2.3% and obesity 14%. By 2023, the type 2 diabetes rate was 15.8%; overweight and obesity was 75%.[59,60,61] At least a third of the patients on any given unit were now diabetic. These were literally heart-stopping numbers.

The second surprise was the sheer number of medications patients were taking. In 1975, we used paper charting, and the average patient's medication record took up only about a quarter of a page with three to five medications. By 2011, when I took students to a hospital unit, electronic medical records would print eight to ten pages of medications for each patient. About half of the medications were used to treat the side effects of their primary medications. Some of these were used to treat preventable harmful lifestyle behaviors and most did not exist when I completed my nursing program.

Obesity is complex because so many factors come into play, such as insufficient funds to buy healthy foods, cultural norms, demanding workloads, and widespread availability of fast foods, among other factors. Despite cardiac surgeries and diagnostic tools saving innumerable lives, the lack of personal responsibility for obesity may lead to the idea that we can "fix" the outcomes of unhealthy lifestyle choices. A cheaper option would be to focus on prevention by avoiding harmful habits and promoting healthy lifestyles. What is missing is the willpower to support healthy living choices. We can't always be in control of our emotions, but if we can tip the scale toward wiser healthy choices, our bodies will reap the benefit.

What does it take to have a healthy lifestyle? Run half a marathon? No, but walk a mile, then gradually work up to a few miles daily. Eat kale and fish? No, but drop an unhealthy food choice each week and replace it with a desirable healthy option. Be deliberate about "cheat" choices. Have one or two chocolate chip cookies; don't finish the bag in one day.

I learned an important lesson as a young nurse. My beloved grandfather was diagnosed with a fatal brain tumor when he was sixty-five and I was twenty-five. He was so upset that he spent the last decade of his life giving up cream in his coffee because of high cholesterol, only to die of cancer. Common sense is key. That way, we don't regret whatever claims our life. Moderation is less restrictive and promotes compliance.

Final Thoughts

I sit in amazement that I was part of this incredible journey. Thinking back to the moon landing that summer day in 1969, the tremendous strides are indeed miraculous. That moment of wonder and ambition ignited an unparalleled era of medical innovation. What began as the pursuit of space exploration would transform medicine and save lives. Little did I realize the Apollo mission would not only inspire me but also propel me into a career where I could contribute to those advancements.

As I look to the future, I hold my breath. Our work isn't done. These innovations are financially fragile. I feel a responsibility to preserve the progress we've made. As we move forward, we must remain vigilant, ensuring that the critical medical research and programs that transformed our lives continue to thrive. We must be mindful to sustain our precious medical miracles so future generations will benefit from the medical advancements we have enjoyed.

About the Author

Dr. Phyllis Heintz is a first-generation college graduate who pursued her dream of becoming a nurse. She holds associate and bachelor's degrees in nursing, a master's in nursing administration with a minor in business administration, and a doctorate in human development, with a concentration in transformative learning for social justice.

Dr. Heintz stood at the bedside for two decades in various critical care settings. She spent the next two decades in executive positions at a small rural hospital and non-profit organizations, including the American Association of Critical-Care Nurses where she served as the executive director of the world's largest specialty nursing organization.

She later joined the faculty of the Department of Nursing at California State University, Bakersfield, in one of California's most medically underserved counties. She served as the department Chair and is now Emeritus faculty. She is a published academic author. Her greatest hope is that by sharing stories of her life and career, others can imagine how their life's goals can be achieved with focus, perseverance, and the unwavering belief one can prevail.

Dr. Heintz can be reached at pheintz@csub.edu

Timeline of Medical Innovations

This timeline captures an astoundingly prolific period for medical innovations.

1940s

1945

- UW School of Nursing formed; Dean Elizabeth Sterling Soule hired founding faculty

1946

- UW School of Medicine formed; Dean Dr. Edward Turner hired founding faculty

1948

- Dr. Robert Williams joins UW SOM as founding Chair of the Department of Medicine

1950s – Research Agendas Established

1958

- Spacelabs is formed to create cardiac monitoring and telemetry systems for NASA

1959

- Dr. Lester Sauvage founds Hope Heart Institute
- Wayne Quinton founds Quinton Instrument Company

1960s – Decade of "Firsts" and Concept Development

1960

- Dr. Belding Scribner and Wayne Quinton developed the Scribner Arteriovenous Shunt
- Dr. Belding Scribner conducts first long-term dialysis treatment
- Wayne Quinton makes the first Teflon shunt at the bedside of a chronic renal failure patient, implanted by Dr. David Dillard of Dr. Scribner's team for the first maintenance dialysis treatment
- CPR developed as a "physician-only" procedure
- Dr. E. Donnall Thomas arrives at UW as a visiting

professor conducts the first bone marrow transplant at the University Hospital.

1961

- Dr. Robert Hickman joined Dr. Belding Scribner's group to develop shunts and catheters for "dialysis and other procedures."

- Dr. Belding Scribner creates and obtains funding for an outpatient dialysis Center

1962

- Seattle Artificial Kidney Center opens; Dr. Christopher Blagg leads the world's first out-of-hospital community-based dialysis center; registered nurses perform dialysis instead of physicians; run in collaboration with King County Medical Society and Dr. James Havilland, President

- The Admissions and Policy Committee of the Seattle Artificial Kidney Center "Dialysis Committee" formed to select patients for time on dialysis machines, foundational for field of Bioethics

1963

- Dr. Lester Sauvage is first surgeon to "successfully substitute a vein for a coronary artery

- Dr. Leonard Cobb appointed Director of Cardiology at Harborview Medical Center, appointed Professor of Medicine
- Dr. E. Donnall Thomas recruited to UW SOM by Department of Medicine Chair, Dr. Robert Williams to establish work in marrow transplantation

1964

- Dr. Belding Scribner and team develop home hemodialysis system for overnight dialysis
- Dr. Henry Tenckhoff recruited by Dr. Scribner to join his group; later developed indwelling peritoneal dialysis catheter and the peritoneal dialysis machine

1965

- CPR reclassified to an "emergency procedure" for doctors, nurses, and ambulance personnel
- Senator Henry Jackson introduces the "first legislation for dialysis and renal treatment"
- Gemini IV space mission uses Spacelabs telemetry to monitor astronaut vital signs during orbit

1968

- Dr. Henry Tenckhoff develops indwelling peritoneal dialysis catheter and the peritoneal dialysis machine
- First ICU and CCU monitoring systems in hospitals developed by Spacelabs

1969

- Dr. Leonard Cobb and Seattle Fire Chief Gordon Vickery co-found Medic One
- Community grant for $450,000 over 3 years funds establish Medic One (first unit nicknamed "Moby Pig")
- Dr. Henry Tenckhoff develops first automated home peritoneal dialysis unit
- Dr. E. Donnall Thomas successfully completed first matched sibling bone marrow transplant for patient with advanced leukemia
- First moon landing by Neil Armstrong using Spacelabs medical telemetry

1970s –Decade of More "Firsts" and Clinical Adoptions

1970

- Medic One program begins

- First EMS 911 system started in King County
- First EMS call
- Seattle Paramedic Program "one of first in the world" established between Harborview Medical Center and University of Washington
- Northwest Kidney Center offers peritoneal dialysis
- Dr. Sherrill Slichter joins Puget Sound Blood Center, improved methods of collecting and storing platelets

1971

- Grassroots community campaign to save Medic One
- Dr. Michael Copass arrives at Harborview Medical Center
- President Richard Nixon declares war on cancer, signs into law the National Cancer Act of 1971

1972

- Medic 2 (CPR training for community) established by Dr. Leonard Cobb
- Dr. Leonard Cobb holds mass CPR training throughout Seattle with 100,000 citizens trained (AHA History of CPR) First in the world

- Dr. Henry Tenckhoff develops first automated peritoneal dialysis machine using reverse osmosis
- Congress passes Medicare End-Stage Renal Disease Program to fund dialysis treatments
- Washington State law changed to eliminate need for direct supervision of paramedics in field

1973

- American Heart Association recommends CPR be taught to public
- Dr. Robert Hickman places first Broviac catheter in leukemia patient
- Dr. Lester Sauvage performs first femoropopliteal graft
- End-Stage Renal Disease patients eligible for Social Security Disability Insurance

1974

- AHA adopts position that emergency cardiac care includes the Chain of Survival
- AHA declares Sudden Cardiac Death a public health crisis
- Burn Center opens at Harborview Medical Center

1975

- Bone Marrow Transplant Program moved to newly created Fred Hutchinson Research Center
- Medic One program expands to train paramedics from other emergency groups in King County

1976

- FDA Medical Device Statute introduced mandating safety and effectiveness of medical devices

1979

- Advanced Cardiac Life Support developed
- First "Fred Hutch patient to receive marrow from unrelated marrow donor to treat leukemia." Led to of national marrow registry

1980s

1981

- King County, WA establishes program for giving instructions to perform CPR over the telephone
- First AIDS case identified as a slow growing blood borne virus

1982

- Airlift Northwest started by Dr. Michael Copass
- HIV epidemic emerges
- Mavis Tsai, PhD completes her doctoral work on therapy for women sexually abused as children.

1986

- AHA calls for a community system for ACLS
- Dr. Sherrill Slichter wins NIH grant to establish national unrelated bone marrow donor registry

1988

- Dr. Richard Cummins promotes "Chain of Survival" concept at Citizen CPR Foundation Conference

1990s

1990

- Dr. E. Donnall Thomas received the Nobel Prize in medicine for pioneering bone marrow transplantation research
- Fred Hutchinson Research Center now world's largest bone marrow transplant unit

1991

- Patient Self-Determination Act passed

1993

- Dr. Leonard Cobb turns directorship of Medic One over to Dr. Michael Copass

1995

- Sarah Sanford, CEO of AACN provides testimony to House subcommittee regarding the importance of funding for AHCPR to create a pilot research project for implementation of Advance Directives

1996

- Gordon Vickery dies of heart failure at 76, Seattle Fire Chief started Medic One with Dr. Leonard Cobb

1998

- Dr. Sherrill Schlicter receives the Karl Landsteiner Memorial Award, the top research honor from the American Association of Blood Banks

2000s

2002

- Dr. Belding Scribner receives Albert Lander Award for Clinical Medical Research, the US equivalent of the Nobel Prize

2003

- Dr. Belding Scribner dies after falling from his houseboat at age 82.

2005

- Dr. Richard Cummins "Honoree for Emergency Cardiovascular Care" by AHA and ILOR as a "Giant of CPR"

2005

- AACN publishes the comprehensive *Acute and Critical Care Choices Guide to Advance Directives*

2007

- Dr. Robert Hickman awarded the UW Medical Alumni Association "Honor Award and Gold Key" to recognize his medical accomplishments and distinguished service to humanity.

2009

- Wayne Quinton awarded Alumnus Summa Laude Dignatus (alumnus worthy of highest praise)

2010s

2010

- Dr. Leonard Cobb honored as 1 of 4 "Pioneers in Paramedicine" Lifetime Achievement Award as a founder of Seattle's Medic One Program
- Dr. Belding Scribner honored in Nephrology Hall of Fame, 50 years after developing the Scribner Shunt

2012

- Dr. Donnall Thomas dies of heart failure at age 92.
- Dr. Richard Olney dies of ALS at age 64.

2015

- Wayne Quinton dies at age 94.
- Dr. Lester Sauvage dies peacefully at age 88.

2017

- Dr. Henry Tenckhoff dies at age 86.

2019

- Dr. Robert Hickman dies peacefully of natural causes at age 92.

2020s

2020

- Dr. Michael Copass named to the EMS Hall of Fame
- COVID-19 vaccine released on an emergency basis
- Dr. Albert Jonsen dies at 89

2023

- A new Golden Age of Medicine declared by the National Institutes of Health.
- Dr. Leonard Cobb dies at age 96 by choosing to use Washington state's Death with Dignity Act to request lethal doses of medication as his body was deteriorating.

2024

- Dr. Michael Copass dies at 86 in a skilled nursing facility following a stroke

2025

- Dr. Sherril Schlicter is 87

- Dr. Richard Cummins is 80

References

1. Anonymous. Spacelabs company history. SpaceLabs Healthcare. December 21, 2017. https://www.spacelabshealthcare.com/about-us/our-heritage

2. Fairman J, Lynaugh J. Critical care nursing: A history. Philadelphia, PA: University of Pennsylvania Press, 1998.

3. Marmor J. Back from the brink. University of Washington Magazine. 2003; Summer, 28-9.

4. Eisenberg, MS. The resuscitation greats: Leonard Cobb and Medic One. Resuscitation. 2002; 54: 5-9.

5. Cobb LA, Alvarez H, Copass, MK. A rapid response system for out-of-hospital cardiac emergencies. *Medical Clinics of North America*. 1976; 60(2): 283-92.

6. Seattle Fire Department. (2010). Medic One program founder Dr. Leonard Cobb honored. *Fireline Blog*. Seattle.gov. http://fireline.seattle.gov/2010/05/12/seattle-fire-depart

ment-%u2019s-medic-one-program

7. Anonymous. In this issue. *Resuscitation*. 2002; 54:1-3.

8. Paramedic Training Program. History of Medic One. *Harborview Medical Center*, 2015.

9. Wikipedia. The Seattle and King County Emergency Medical Services System. 2019.

10. Schwartz P. Training of nurses is moving from hospitals into colleges. *The New York Times*, 1972. March 26; 76.

11. Hope Heart Institute. Our history. February 14, 2018. http://hopeheart.org/about/

12. Aleccia J. Dr. Lester R. Sauvage, Seattle heart surgeon, dies at 88. *Seattle Times*. 2015. https://www.seattletimes.com/seattle-news/obituaries/dr-lester-sauvage-seattle-heart-surgeon-dies-at-88

13. Dubois C. Prayer: It's just what the doctor ordered. *U.S. Catholic*. 1997; October: 25-30.

14. Anonymous. Our Founder. *Hope Heart Institute.* 2018. http://www.hopeheart.org/about/ourfounder

15. Cousler WG. In memoriam: Belding H. Scribner, M.D. *Kidney International*. 2003; 64: 1155-56.

16. Blagg CR. Belding Hibbard Scribner—better known as Scrib. *Clinical Journal of the American Society of Nephrology.* 2010; 5(12): 2146–49. https://doi.org/10.2215/cjn.07640810

17. Wills A, Bolcer JD. Campus history. *University of Washington.* Charleston, SC: Arcadia Publishers. 2014.

18. Jonsen AR. The God Squad and the origins of transplantation ethics and policy. *Journal of Law, Medicine, and Ethics*. 2007; Summer: 238-40.

19. Alexander S. They decide who lives, who dies: Medical miracle puts a moral burden on a small committee. *Life*. 1962; 102-104, 106, 108, 110, 115, 117, 118, 123, 124, 127.

20. Scribner BH. Medical dilemmas: The old is new. *Nature Medicine*. 2002; 8: 1066-67.

21. Butler C.R., Mehrotra R., Tonelli MR, Lam DY The evolving ethics of dialysis in the United States: A principlist bioethics approach. *Clinical Journal of Society of Nephrology*. 2016; 11(4): 704-709.

22. Anonymous. Albert "Al" Rupert Jonsen, PhD. *University of Washington Medicine.* 2020.

23. Lenzer J. Belding Scribner. *British Medical Journal*. 2003;

July: 167.

24. Garner J. (2015). Wayne Quinton, UW's Wayne Quinton, 1921-2015. *University of Washington Magazine.* March 1, 2015. https://magazine.washington.edu/wayne-quinton-1921-2015/

25. Szeto CC, Todd SI, Philip KTL. In Memorium of Henry Tenckhoff. *Artificial Organs*. 2017; 41(8): 697-99.

26. Anonymous. (2017). Peritoneal dialysis pioneer dies. *UW News*, March 27, 2017. https://medicine.uw.edu/news/peritoneal-dialysis-pioneer-dies

27. Anonymous. Father of bone marrow transplantation Dr. E. Donnall Thomas dies. *Fred Hutch Cancer Center*. October 20, 2012. Father of bone marrow transplantation Dr. E. Donnall Thomas dies | Fred Hutchinson Cancer Center

28. Thomas ED. E. Donnall Thomas – Biographical. *Nobel Prize.org*. 1990 https://www.nobelprize.org/nobel_prizes/medicine/laureates/1990

29. Anonymous. Childhood Cancer Statistics. *American Childhood Cancer Association* (ACCO). 2018

30. Kolata G. 2 American transplant pioneers win Nobel Prize in Medicine. *New York Times*, October 9, 1990.

31. Medical Alumni Association. Alumnus profile: Robert O. Hickman '57. *University of Maryland*, Spring 2007. MAA - Spring 2007 - Robert O. Hickman, '57

32. Broberg B. Blood bank ratchets up research role. *Puget Sound Business Journal.* 2004; 24:33.

33. National Institute of Medicine. Grantome.com/grant/NIM/P60-HL033775-05. *National Institute of Medicine.*

34. Slichter S.J. Platelet transfusions as replacement therapy. *Triangle.* 1993. 32(2):71-84.

35. Richey J. Airlift Northwest. *Air Medical Association Journal*. 2012. 06(14): 215.

36. Anonymous. Harborview legend Michael Copass begins leadership transition. *UW News*. November 20, 2008. http://www.washington.edu/news/2008/11/20/harborview-legend-michael-copass-begins-leadership-transition/

37. Seattle Fire Department. Medic One program founder Dr. Leonard Cobb honored. *Fireline Blog*. Seattle.gov. 2010.

http://fireline.seattle.gov/2010/05/12/seattle-fire-department-%u2019s-medic-one-program

38. Poppy J. Seattle to the rescue. *Health*. 1990.6: 69.

39. Goodrich C. Nursing in flight. *American Association of Critical-Care Nurses.* 2022. www.aacn.org/nursing-excellence/nurse-stories/nursing-in-flight

40. Cummins R. Emergency medical services and sudden cardiac arrest with the chain of survival concept. *Annu. Rev. Publ. Health.* 1993. 14:313-33.

41. Anonymous. Cummins joins 'Giants of CPR.' *UW News.* 2005. February 25. http://www.washington.edu/news/2005/02/24/cummins-joins-giants-of-cpr/

42. Brody JE. Why so many die needlessly: Broken rescue chain. *New York Times.* 1994. Why So Many Die Needlessly: Broken Cardiac Rescue Chain - The New York Times

43. Greenleaf RK, Spears LC, Covey SR, Senge PM. *Servant leadership: A journey into the nature of legitimate power and greatness.* Paulist Press; 2002.

44. McFadden RD. Karen Ann Quinlan, 31, dies; Focus of

'76 right to die case. *The New York Times*. 1985. June 12.

45. Lewin T. Nancy Cruzan dies, outlived by a debate over the right to die. *The New York Times.* 1990. December 27.

46. ALS Association. Dr. Richard K. Olney, founding director of the ALS Center at UCSF, dies after eight-year battle with Lou Gehrig's Disease. *ALS News.* 2012. January 30. http://webgw.alsa.org/site/PageServer?pagename=GW_9_in_the_news_2012_01_30_Dr_Richard_Olney_Remembered&printer_friendly=1

47. Anonymous. Seer database for cancer statistics 1975 to 2022. *National Cancer Institute*. 2022. SEER*Stat Databases: SEER November 2022 Submission

48. Heintz (Reading) PA. *Dimensions of organizational cultural diversity for lesbian executives.* Seminar session presented at the Sixth Annual International Critical and Feminist Perspectives in Nursing Conference: Personal Journeys and the Politics of Difference. Carlow College, Prout's Neck, Maine.1995.

49. Heintz PA. *Identities at the intersections.* (Unpublished doctoral dissertation). *Fielding Graduate University.* 2009.

50. Wing Sue D. Microaggressions: Death by a thousand cuts.

Scientific American. 2021. March 30.

51. Heintz PA. Work-life dilemmas emerging from lesbian executives' narratives. *Career Development Quarterly*. 2012. *60*, 122-133.

52. Heintz PA. *The balancing act: Preserving personal authenticity in the workplace.* Podium session presented at the Out & Equal Workplace National Summit. 2010. October.

53. Heintz PA. *The silver tsunami: A glimpse inside the wave.* Podium session presented at the Robert and Edith Cochran Annual Gerontological Lecture. 2014. March.

54. Spencer K. *12 lessons.* Katherin Spencer Publishing; 2012.

55. Benner P. *From novice to expert: Excellence and power in clinical nursing practice.* Prentice Hall; 2001.

56. University of Wisconsin Population Health Initiative. County health rankings and roadmaps: 2022 state report California. *University of Wisconsin School of Medicine and Public Health*. 2022. www.countyhealthrankings.org

57. Eiseley LC. *The star thrower.* Times Books; 1978.

58. Fox CS, Pencina MJ, Meigs JB, Ramachandran SV, Yamini SL, D'Agostino RB. Trends

in the incidence of Type 2 Diabetes Mellitus from the 1970s to the 1990s: The Framingham Heart Study. *Circulation.* 2006; 113(25). https://doi.org/10.1161/Circulationaha.106.613828

59. Anonymous. United States: COVID-19 weekly death Rate by vaccination status. *Centers for Disease Control and Prevention*. 2003. https://www.ourworldindata.org

60. Anonymous. National Diabetes Statistics Report, Diabetes. *Centers for Disease Control.* 2024. May 15. https://www.cdc.gov/diabetes/php/data-research/index.html

61. Agrawal N. Three quarters of U.S. adults are now overweight or obese. *New York Times.* 2024. Three-Quarters of U.S. Adults Are Now Overweight or Obese - The New York Times

62. Anonymous. Life expectancy in the US declines a year and a half in 2020. *Centers for Disease Control and Prevention.* Retrieved December 4, 2021. https://www.cdc.gov/nchs/pressroom/nchs_press_releases/2021/202107.html

63. Wallace-Wells D. Suddenly, it looks like we're in a golden age for medicine. *New York Times Magazine.* 2023; June 23.

64. Jonson CK. Next Big Advance in Cancer Treatment Could Be a Vaccine. *The Seattle Times*. 2023; June 27.

Made in the USA
Middletown, DE
01 August 2025

11514349R00151